Pick It
and
Flick It

You are such an inspiration!
You shall come forth as gold.

Holly Johnson

Psalm 91:11
Zep 3:17

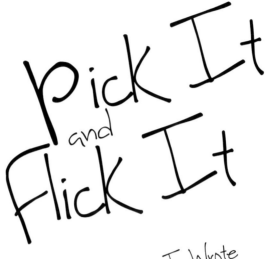

Pick It and Flick It

The Prescription I Wrote for My Healing

Rx by: Holly Johnson, M.D.

TATE PUBLISHING
AND ENTERPRISES, LLC

Published by Tate Publishing & Enterprises, LLC
127 E. Trade Center Terrace | Mustang, Oklahoma 73064 USA
1.888.361.9473 | www.tatepublishing.com

Tate Publishing is committed to excellence in the publishing industry. The company reflects the philosophy established by the founders, based on Psalm 68:11,
"The Lord gave the word and great was the company of those who published it."

Book design copyright © 2013 by Tate Publishing, LLC. All rights reserved.
Author photo by Spencer Freeman
Cover design by Rodrigo Adolfo
Interior design by Jake Muelle

Published in the United States of America

ISBN: 978-1-62510-809-8
1. Health & Fitness / Diseases / Cancer
2. Health & Fitness / Healing
13.07.02

Praises for Pick It and Flick It

"As a coach, I would certainly want someone with Holly's winning spirit on my team."

Coach Ara Parseghian, former head coach of Miami University, Northwestern University, and the University of Notre Dame, College Football Hall of Fame inductee, and founder of the Ara Parseghian Medical Research Foundation

"I was prepared to like this book because I already loved and admired the author. But I was not prepared to be so engaged that I was brought to laughter, tears, and worship. God has all of us go through what one of us does, so that we are brought closer to Him and to each other. Thank you for your story Holly, one that prepares us to go through our own struggles in the future!"

Dr. Joel C. Hunter, Senior Pastor of Northland Community Church–A Church Distributed, spiritual advisor to the President of the United States, and author of *Interstate 80: Your Journey on the Highway*, *A New Kind of Conservative*, and *Church Distributed*.

Dedication

For all beloved cancer fighters, cancer crushers, cancer survivors, and their loved ones. It is also written in honor of those who have been healed but in an eternal way. "But he knows the way that I take; when he has tested me, I will come forth as gold" (Job 23:10, NIV).

Acknowledgments

To my chemo posse—MaryAnne, Karen, Zeddy, Donna and to those unnamed who shared the chairs every two weeks—thank you for encouraging me, for sharing your stories, and for saving the seat next to the bathroom for me. To my Army of Angels, thank you for reading my story as it was happening and now again as we pray for the cure. You are my own heart walking around outside of my body. To Dr. Bob Reynolds, thank you for saving my life and for healing me in more ways than you will ever know. To Katina, my waterhead of a nurse and sister in Christ, you, as well as He, were my rock and my salvation (Psalm 62). To my Ya-Ya sisters, thank you for going up the river and down the river with me along this crazy ride. You know my soul. To Nancy and Tiffany, maybe I could have done this without you, but I certainly would not have wanted to. "Thank you" is not ever going to be enough for what you have given; you are the best a girl could ever hope for. To Melissa, my partner in crime to get this book written! I am better for knowing you and having you as a friend and editor. Thank you for hours of pouring over copy and fixing my mistakes. "You is kind. You is smart. You is important." To Mom, thank you for loving me as only a mother can and for making me write my English papers over and over. To Eric, my baby , thank you for the inspiration for title ideas, for g in me, and for knowing what to say and what not to say at the all the right moments. How do you do that? To Tate Publishing, thank you for taking a chance on me so I could tell my story. To Griffin, thank you for the love in a Biscuit. To my workmates, thank you for listening to hours of first drafts and for telling me when to eat and when to sit down and for your amazing support in helping me to Livestrong every day as we do what we do best—caring for the sick and injured. To Herdley, thank you for hours of listening to me bare my soul. You are a blessing. To Dr. Hunter, thank you for rallying around me in my time of deepest need and hurt and for the healing of anointment. To Shane, my hubby, thank you for being my right-hand man, not just yesterday and today, but always. Thank you, God, the Great Physician and My Healer, for answered prayers and for making this storytelling possible.

Table of Contents

The Elephant in My Chest

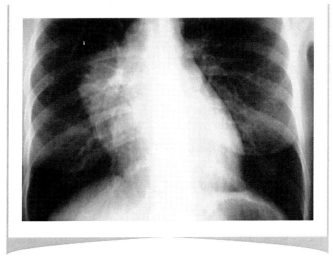

Photo by the author

My abnormal chest x-ray. The white mass on your left is not supposed to be there.

RX: Listen to your body, and no matter who you are, or what you do, or how busy you are, seek help during times such as this.

I am a doctor. I diagnose illness and disease every day. I help sick and injured people and talk to them about how to heal and how to try to live their best life. Frequently patients come to me with a cough, and I diagnose them with things like bronchitis, pneumonia, postnasal drip, or allergies. In March, I had a cough too. It was a dry cough, and it had lasted for two and a half months seemingly triggered by an overwhelming apple-cinnamon plug-in air freshener at work. Even once I begged my coworkers to remove the air freshener, however, the cough persisted. It was triggered by other smelly things too, like fruity body lotions, tuna sandwiches, cigarette smoke, other people's breath, and by air-conditioning.

I was in great physical shape. I ran ten miles a week, biked the trail, and trained with weights. I worked full time, balanced my free time with my husband and friends, and went to church on Sundays.

I remember thinking that this felt weird. I wasn't sick! I was healthy, and I had always taken good care of myself. I exercised, I ate healthy foods; I even ate an apple a day! I got my routine physicals and blood work. Nothing was wrong with me except for this inexplicable cough! I coughed for over two months until finally I couldn't take it anymore. It came to the point where I literally couldn't stand up or sit up without coughing.

I slumped in a chair one Friday night at work in between seeing a patient with an ear infection and one with a broken finger, and I turned to my x-ray technician and said, "Would you mind taking a chest x-ray on me? I want to make sure I don't have pneumonia!"

Expecting to see nothing and hoping I would just make an appointment with a pulmonologist, a lung specialist, within the next week, I walked into the dark room with its spooky shadows and fluorescent light boxes. With a delicious cracking noise, I snapped my x-ray films into the light. I stood and stared, alone, aghast at what I saw. I saw something I have never seen on anyone's x-ray.

There was a huge white, well-defined mass in my chest extending from the right side of my heart. I thought to myself, *What the heck is that?* I stood alone in the dark, my head spinning, and I felt that I was about to live someone else's life and certainly not my own. I had a mass in my chest. There, I said it. It's what many people would consider the elephant in the room. I didn't want an elephant in my room or in my chest for that matter! A new reality was set in motion. My life changed in that instant.

At work, I showed my nurses the x-ray. No one quite knew what to say to me after that although one of them asked me, "Are you scared?"

I replied, "I don't know yet."

Facing my own mortality and vulnerability, however, I did know one thing. I had a decision to make. I could pout and feel like my life was nearly over, or I could fight with a punch of grace and a hit of humor. It was sink or swim.

I was stunned and had to finish work that day and then go home to tell my husband. I drove home in a daze, not even sure if I stopped at all the traffic lights. When I got home, I immediately sat down with my husband on our khaki-green oversized couch and told him about the elephant. Somehow we got through the night and the weekend without completely falling apart.

A few days later, a radiologist called me at home. Never a good sign. He asked me why I ordered my own chest x-ray. I talked to him about the cough and how I couldn't sit up straight without the cough jolting me for a breath. He told me it could be one of many benign things like my thymus, a cyst of some kind, or a noncancerous tumor. He also told me that it could be something malignant like a lymphoma. Once my own fears were confirmed that my chest x-ray was definitely not normal, my mind went racing...This journey was only beginning. I thought to myself, *Welcome to my temporary new life. Get ready to swim!*

In order to diagnose and to see the elephant in my chest in better detail, four days after I took that chest x-ray I was lying face up in a CT machine breathing in, holding my breath, exhaling, and imagining that this was all a mistake. The CT machine table was flat and hard, and as short as I am my feet felt like they were hanging off the end. My arms were extended above my head, and I was looking at this giant diagnostic circle that would capture images of the tumor inside of me. I heard it purring, warming up to me and my situation as it had countless times before me...capturing images of so many others. This marvelous medical machine had witnessed countless feelings of anxiety, sadness, and worry. It could witness and feel the weight of all that but could not absorb those feelings for any of us and take them away for us.

In the machine, I looked overhead at two Pac-Man–like faces. One on the left was green and its mouth was open, and even though the corners of the lips were upturned, the silhouette of the face wasn't necessarily smiling at me either. It was encouraging me to just breathe. The face on the right was red, and its mouth was closed. Its cheeks looked puffed out, and when it flashed red, I was supposed to hold my breath and stop breathing. The contrast dye for the CT was pushed into my left inner elbow vein and my arm was suddenly gripped in pain. I had a warm sensation in my bladder. I felt like I had just peed in my pants! I held my breath and then the procedure was over. The IV was taken out of my arm, high fives were shared with the CT techs, and I was back in the waiting room, awaiting my fate. This could be the defining moment...The elephant could have a name.

Not Your Mother's Suntan Oil

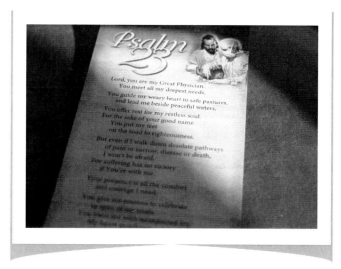

Photo by the author

A version of Psalm 23 that carried me through my healing.
"Your presence is all the comfort and courage I need."

RX: Believe you will be healed, and get anointed.

There are five forms of healing. I believe in every single one of them…and I will not hesitate to capitalize on each of them if it means well-being, health, rest, and peace for me or for my patients. I learned about the five forms of healing from an elder at my church. His name is Peter, and I call him Tall Peter because he stands at about six feet five inches tall. He towers over us all! He is one of the best huggers on the planet, and as big and tall as he is, his hugs are one size fits all. Tall Peter, my husband, Shane, and I got into a discussion about the five different ways of healing; we also agreed that all healing comes from God in one way or another.

The first form of healing is instantaneous healing. The concept of instantaneous healing doesn't need much explanation, yet it is an inexplicable event. This happens when there is clearly a divine intervention, and we witness what is known as a miracle. Nothing else can explain this type of healing. Miracles certainly do not happen often enough, but they do happen from time to time.

The second way we can be healed is through our own immune systems. God created, designed, and built our bodies and that includes every cell in our immune systems, which helps us to fend off viruses, bacteria, diseases, and sometimes even cancerous cells. Our immune system includes everything from our first line of visible defense known as our skin, to microscopic white blood cells, which work to destroy foreign cells that would otherwise create illness.

Another type of healing comes from physicians and health care teams who work as an extension of the hand of God. They are given wisdom from God through their education and studies. They apply their knowledge, operate to remove disease, and listen to many symptoms and hearts in order to give the best possible outcomes. They prescribe medications such as antibiotics, chemotherapy, and vaccinations. These pills, elixirs, and injections are created by scientists and researchers through the love of God to ultimately help our bodies fight off or prevent disease.

A shift in our attitudes and emotions toward a healthier outlook is the fourth form of healing. This form of healing is often the most difficult as it requires intentional, focused effort on our part. Yes, we have to work in order to heal—it's not all going to be handed to us on a silver platter! It involves letting go of past hurts, adopting an attitude of forgiveness, and purposefully seeking and finding joy. It means setting boundaries and getting rid of stress or learning how to manage it differently. Shifting our attitude means mindfully putting aside anger, regret, resentment, despair, and hopelessness to make room for more positive emotions. No one can do this for us. The old adage is true, "If it is to be, it is up to me!"

Finally, the last form of healing is called perfect healing. This is found in heaven where there is no disease, no cancer, no pain, no depression. Perfect healing is where healing is complete.

Being healed doesn't necessarily mean that illness goes away, but it does mean finding health, joy, peace, and light even in the darkness that surrounds us. The trials that rain upon us as we slosh through the storms toward healing, and hopefully cure, beget perseverance. Perseverance builds character. Character, in turn, creates hope. The minute I saw my chest x-ray with the tumor staring me down, I started to grow in all of these areas. I decided to not quit, to not give up, to not give in, to not let my disease beat me. I decided I would persevere as long as it took. I wanted to develop my character as a woman of faith. I wanted to be more patient, more human, more real, more in tune with others and our common denominators of suffering, fear, stress, and anxiety. I wanted to then rise above these denominators and see hope—stare it down in the eye—and more than anything, I wanted to be healed.

One of the first words of advice I received after I saw the tumor was to be anointed with oil as soon as possible. I believe in divine intervention as a form of healing. I wanted all the prayer I could gather. Before my surgery, before my diagnosis, before I even imagined the worst or best possible outcome, I called my church and asked to be anointed. I decided to pray for and ask for the impossible. I wanted a miracle, and I wanted the senior pastor: difficult requests to have granted in a church with twelve thousand worshippers! Instead, I was told that an associate pastor and two elders would be available and to keep praying for that miracle. The anointing date was set.

The day before we met with the surgeon for the first time, my husband, my mom, my best friend, and I met in the church lobby. An associate pastor met us and led us to a prayer room. We were introduced to two elders: Tall Peter and Dan. The room had a dark-colored couch and several chairs surrounding a low, long, black table. There was a lone box of pop-up Kleenex tissues on the table. Expecting that the associate pastor or one of the elders would be anointing me, I sat down on the couch and waited for instructions. Then, unexpectedly, our senior pastor walked into the room! Shane told me that I gasped as I stood up and walked toward Pastor Hunter. He hugged me and whispered, "God has you." I looked him in his hopeful blue eyes. I saw care, compassion, immersion in my moment of hurt; and I saw a glimpse of Jesus. I felt like I was breathing in a pool made of velvet as I shared my story and as Tall Peter read from James chapter five.

I sat in one of the chairs with this close circle of angels around me. Pastor Hunter stood in front of me and dipped his right index finger in a small pot of oil. His light touch crossed my forehead as the slippery anointing oil nourished my skin, and I was blessed in the name of the Father, the Son, and the Holy Spirit. Hands were laid on me as I submitted to the power of prayer and the moment. I closed my eyes. I felt hands lightly rubbing my head, scratching my back, and touching my right shoulder. I even felt a glowing, intense warmth from the hand on my shoulder.

I was placed in the hold of God, the greatest Physician, the ultimate Healer. The prayer for me was that God perform a miracle and simply take the tumor away as only He is able to do. The prayer continued that if that was not God's will to make a miracle out of me, that I would be healed through the hands of the surgeon and other physicians that would surround me on this journey. I was feeling the power of His spirit, and as tears rained down my face, I cried out loud, "I believe! I believe!" I remember thinking to myself, *I believe, Lord, that you have blessed my path. You knew me before I was born and knew that this moment would come. I feel you. I see you. Hold me in your hands. I confess my belief that you will heal me and carry me as I walk down this road.*

Then, it was over. I felt lighter. My chest felt lighter. I was no longer breathing under velvet water. On the way out, I overheard one of the pastors say to my husband, "You have a very healthy wife." That "sealed the heal" for me.

This powerful spiritual experience was certainly not anything like slathering on my mother's suntan oil, ready to bake in the sun, and getting burned to a crispy red color. Instead, in those simple words, in those intense prayer moments, in the heat of the hand on my shoulder, in the oil that was streaked across my forehead, I had no doubt that I was not going to be burned to a crisp. Rather, I was already healing.

Grace in the Bathroom

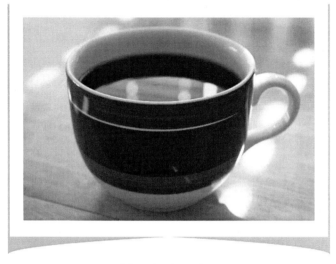

Photo by the author

When I'm in hot water, I become more of who I already am.

RX: Seek grace. You may find
it in the strangest places.

Sunday, two days before my surgery, there was no doubt about where I wanted to start my week... at church. I was seeking spiritual solace, peace, hope, and emotional strength. I wanted to forget about the journey I was about to travel on even if my memory could get lost for just an hour. We attend a large church called Northland: A Church Distributed, which has concurrent worship services at several sites across Central Florida and via web stream. We have known our pastor for over a decade and had, in a matter of days, become closer to him in spirit because of my anointing experience. I don't think that he had anything special planned for me that week, and I doubt that he changed his sermon based on whom he blessed or anointed the week before, but strangely, here is what happened that Sunday morning and where I found grace.

As I sat slumped in the church's blue, cloth-covered pew seat so that I wouldn't cough, I was flanked by my mother and my husband, cautiously watching my every move. The church grew dark and quiet as the overhead screen came to life and music of "Ode to Joy" and "God of Wonders" played in the background. The worship leader led us in prayer. She said,

> Lord, you created everything we see and everything we don't see...We look at this world and sometimes it makes us feel very small, and sometimes we are reminded of how weak and fragile we are, yet we are thankful. Jesus also lived in a body that wouldn't always cooperate, and He understands our suffering...Thank you, God, for the grace you want to shed on us.

Then, there was a video of a pretty young woman, in her late twenties, who started to speak on the screen. She had long dark hair and a friendly smile. She started to tell her story of pain and suffering and her uncooperative body. Three years prior, she was not feeling well and was having chest discomfort and fatigue. She made an appointment with her family doctor. He thought it was probably heartburn, gave her some samples of antacids, and sent her home. The next day, she felt worse, and her mother encouraged her to go back to her doctor's office. She did. A chest x-ray was done, and a photo of that x-ray was then sprawled across the big screen at church for us to see. I about fell out of my seat when I saw a mirror image of my own chest x-ray. She had a tumor in her chest that looked just like mine!

She went on to say that she was ultimately diagnosed with Hodgkin's lymphoma and had to undergo grueling chemotherapy and radiation treatment to overcome it. Photos of her as she lost her hair and she became thin and worn down were shown on the screen. As she suffered with sickness, and persevered through her treatments, she became discouraged when it was time for a body scan, and her cancer was not gone yet. She started to question whether or not heaven was real and whether or not Jesus still loved her. She thought to herself, "This is suffering. Am I going to die? Am I going to heaven?" It took a lot longer than her doctor told her it would take for her to get better. She ultimately held on to hope, and in that hope and with time, her tumor went away and she got better. She went into remission, yet still to this day, she hasn't had a day go by when she hasn't thought about her suffering, her cancer, and what she went through to shake it off. She had lost more than she thought she would lose because of her illness. During the fight for her life, her faith felt like it was destroyed; she had no work, she lost a boyfriend, and she had no hope for the future. Yet when her cancer was gone, she took a deep breath and a long look at herself and said, "That was hard, but I'm still all right!"

Then, the screen went blank, and the church grew dark again. Guess what happened as the lights came back on? She walked out on stage, long hair flowing, healthy, cancer free, and she sang a song. She stood strong in her black shirt with white polka dots and blue jeans, and she was accompanied by a young man on guitar. And the woman in my mirror sang these words: "Why this road? Why this way? I don't have to understand, to believe. You know how far I must go, to see…why this road."

If God is good, why is there suffering? That was the question that our pastor, Dr. Joel Hunter, set out to try to answer that Sunday morning. Here I was in church, trying not to cough as the fireworks were going off in my chest, and visions of my future were falling into my lap like ashes from heaven. The pastor walked out on stage with a yellow shirt, striped tie, and dark suit that fit like a glove. His gray hairs were neatly combed, and his eyes were serious yet twinkling. He started his sermon with prayer.

> Lord, our hurt is holy ground. It is where You
> meet us, and although darkness is the limitation
> of our sight, it is not the absence of Your love.
> Though our minds are vacant of answers, our
> hearts are not left alone.

Our pastor believes that God uses our suffering for redemption, and as we go through hard times, if we get answers to our questions too quickly, we may be glossing over and somehow diminishing why God put us on this planet to begin with. If our prayers are answered immediately or our questions are answered on point, we cannot become the person we were meant to be or have the faith we need to have. Evil comes because there is an evil one; and in the midst of evil and suffering, it is possible to cling to God and be more grateful to Him for His grace and what He has given us.

Unluckily, sometimes we may have no choice of the hurtful circumstances we face, but luckily, we do have a choice of responses when we are faced with the worst— when we are in hot water. Pastor Hunter loves to tell a story about bringing three pots of water to boil. In one pot, he says, imagine throwing in carrots. In the second pot, gently place some eggs, and in the last pot, imagine putting in coffee beans. Let all three pots boil for quite some time. What do you think happens to the carrots? Placed in hot water for a long time, carrots become mushy, wimpy, and limp. And what about the eggs? They become hard-boiled…strong. But what about the coffee beans? Well, they become…coffee. In boiling water, coffee becomes more of what it was intended to become in the first place. The beans unleash their potential, and their full-bodied flavor infiltrates the hot water and makes it whole. When people are in hot water, if we make the choice to be like coffee, the best in us can be brought out that was there all along; and as a result, we have more to offer to others in the form of generosity in action called grace.

Even though I couldn't stand the smell of coffee with my newly sensitive nose and lungs, I wanted to become nothing less than coffee after hearing that story! My choice was made. I wanted to be like Job who says, "But He knows the way that I take; when He has tested me, I will come forth as gold" (Job 23:10). In this moment of my body not cooperating, in this moment of not understanding the unseen, I thought to myself, *I will brew like coffee. I will be patient. I will cling to God. There are results that must come from my suffering. There is gold. And from then on, that became my motto—that even though I was being put to the test, I would come forth as gold.*

As I thought about Job and the grace of God, I was caught off guard when the pastor started to share with the congregation that there was a physician in the church who had a cough for a couple of months and took her own chest x-ray and saw a mass. He was talking about me! He said that I was a woman of faith, obedient to God, and that when I saw the mass, I knew immediately what to do. I called upon the elders of the church to pray for me and to be anointed with oil for healing. Three nights prior to Sunday's service, the elders, my family and friends, and he all laid their hands on me and prayed. He said that he knew I was unnerved, but being a physician, did the congregation think that I would be a better physician because of this suffering or a worse one? He answered the question himself, "Absolutely, a better one, of course! Because she knows what it is like to be helpless. She knows what it is like to lie in a hospital bed and wait for results of a test. She knows what it is like to need encouragement and warmth and not just clinical information. She knows what it is like because she suffered herself." He also said, "I have to believe she will be healed, and because of this, she will become a better healer herself." Outside of our own suffering, he said that there is a bigger picture. He reminded us that evil will come and try to throw us off course, but God will never forsake us and will always love us. He will shed His grace upon us in one form or another. Believe it or not, something good will come out of our suffering—more good than if we never had it.

After the service, I was mentally and emotionally exhausted and needed to use the restroom. As I trudged across the brown tile floor toward the bathroom sinks, coughing, I was compelled to turn and look at the women in line. It was here that I found Grace. Dr. Grace is a well-loved OB/GYN in private practice whom I met in residency. She is an Indian woman with wavy dark hair and kind brown eyes behind wire-rimmed glasses. In greeting me, we held hands, and she asked me how I was doing. I cried and said, "Not too well. Do you remember Pastor Hunter talking about a woman physician in our church with a tumor in her chest?"

"Yes," answered Grace.

"Well, that woman is me," I said through tears.

"Oh, Holly!" Grace exclaimed. "You don't have cancer! Do you?"

And then she started to pray. In the middle of the women's room, toilets flushing, sinks running, and paper towels landing on the floor, she met me where I was and gave me grace when I needed it. She held my hands, she prayed out loud, and she gave me her phone number. Not only did I find Grace in the bathroom, but now I could scroll through my contact list and simply call for Grace whenever I needed it.

Cracked Open

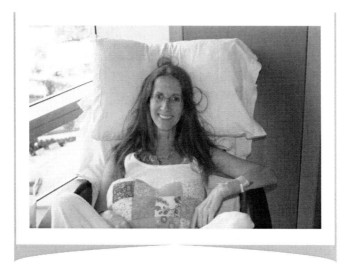

Photo by Shane Johnson

Two days post-op in the hospital with
my healing heart pillow.

RX: Trust in the Chief of Staff.
Fight with a hit of humor.

May 22 was a day that will forever be etched in my memory. At noon that day, Shane, my mother, and I went to my thoracic surgeon's office. It was comfortable there. The waiting room was big and lofty with a lot of windows. The afternoon sunshine streamed in between the slats of the blinds. There was a large, tall, round, dark wood footed table in the center of the room with a huge centerpiece and magazines; and on one wall was one of my favorite paintings called *The Chief of Staff*. I often think of this picture when I am working—as the doctor—and I am trying to figure out the right diagnosis, appropriate treatment, or the right words to talk with a patient.

The Chief of Staff painting is a scene in a calm, dimly lit operating room. The operating room staff, in their blue scrubs, masks, gowns, and gloves is focused on the patient before them; the sterile field is illuminated under a single bright light. The surgeon has a hemostat clutched in his right hand. He is confident with caring, patient eyes. Looking to the left in the painting, I understand why in the midst of life and death, with someone's loved one split open in front of him, the surgeon has this calm peace about him—on his right side stands Jesus. Jesus is looking intently down on the OR field and the surgeon's hands. Jesus has his left arm draped around the surgeon's shoulder. His right hand is inches from the surgeon's, cupping and guiding his hand—every slice, every cauterization, every suture.

In the surgeon's office—as the patient—I couldn't keep my eyes off *The Chief of Staff*. I saw it in a different light than I've seen it before. I saw all of Jesus and none of me. I, the doctor, was shoved under the sterile paper of an operating field, diminished to someone covered in blue garb to match the OR, and I was cracked open as the surgeon and My Chief of Staff went to work on me.

I snapped out of it as my name was called. My mom and Shane followed me as I followed the nurse to a small conference room, and the physician's assistant knocked on the door. Shane was seated on my left, and my mom was seated on my right. I nervously fingered my list of questions I had written on a yellow notepad. The PA had a caring demeanor about him. He was tall, confident, but not excessively so, with sandy-brown hair and blue eyes and a kind smile. He took his time with us, and clearly there was no rush in his pace. I appreciated that. He explained that in order for them to get to the tumor, I would have a sternotomy. This meant that they would make an incision right down the center of my chest, then saw open my breastbone, and pull me open to remove the mass. This was a huge blow to my previous thoughts and wishes. The reality of having a sternotomy, like open-heart patients have, sank in like heavy water weighing down a bowing, weak tarp. You see, I thought that they would have to only minimally move some ribs and that I would have a small scar. Feeling the tears brimming in my eyes, I tried to set aside the fear and disappointment. In a flash, I was reminded that I was not in control, but My Chief of Staff was.

The PA told us that I would come out of surgery with tubes in my chest and that I would be in the intensive care unit for a day. By day two or three, the tubes would come out and then I would be on my way home after day three or four. I wouldn't be able to drive for two to three weeks, and full recovery would take six to eight weeks. While I was in surgery still unconscious and splayed open, the surgeon would take my tumor, the elephant in my chest, to the pathology lab where a frozen section would be done. My tumor margins would be studied, and by the time the surgeon returned to the OR, he would know with 80 percent certainty what my diagnosis was. The PA then asked us what questions we had. I went through my carefully thought out list on my yellow pad, and then thought of one more question. I looked at the PA, and bluntly asked, "Are you a Christian?"

He said, "Yes. Yes, I am."

The Chief of Staff was with me. The painting was for real.

Then, the surgeon entered the room. He immediately met my eye and surprised me by saying, "Hey, I know you! I remember you!" He had met hundreds of residents at Florida Hospital over the years, and for some reason, he remembered me! I stood up, and he hugged me. Then I introduced my husband and my mom, and he hugged them too! We all sat, and my nervous heart started beating away. I could immediately sense the command and confidence in the surgeon's presence. This man, whom I had just met again, personally cared about me. That much was obvious.

At that point, even though I had been carrying around my chest CT scan for three days like a new appendage, I had not felt emotionally strong enough to look at it. With the surgeon in charge, I felt ready to face it. We were led to a light box, and instantly I was face-to-face with my tumor. A five-year-old could have recognized it as an abnormal scan! There it was, at the core of me, sitting in front of and to the right of my heart…a tumor…huge and looming pressed in the mediastinal space between my vital organs yet (luckily) not choking any of them. I saw two bright lymph nodes next to the mass. I prayed then and there—as I dared it to go away—that it was a benign tumor staring back at me.

Back in the conference room, the surgeon was still fifty-fifty whether he thought it was benign or malignant, but everything seemed to be pointing in favor of a benign tumor called a thymoma. He knew that I was healthy, and he assured me that my physical recovery would be fine. He stated that he would take out the whole tumor and possibly a section of lung if the two tissue planes were adhered to one another. He said that my surgical scar would be six inches long—a visual reminder that life is hard, but God is good. Like I asked the PA, I asked my surgeon the same question, "Are you a Christian?"

As he pointed skyward, he replied, "Yes, I am a Christian. I work for Him."

Then, things seemed to start moving really fast for me, and before I knew it, I was a topic of conversation between my surgeon and another physician—the man who would become my oncologist, Dr. Robert Reynolds. The oncologist recommended a CT of my abdomen to make sure there was not a second tumor below my chest. With many phone calls made, paperwork filled out, and a surgery date set, we were whisked off to the imaging site. I drank down two big Styrofoam cups of apricot-orange-colored fluid to drink, and then I was sent over to the hospital for preadmission testing.

I felt bleary-eyed, the world buzzing around me as I was trying to process what was happening to me. I remember telling myself to wake up! I wanted to remember and to deeply feel each moment. I filled out more paperwork and paid my co-pays. I had blood work taken, had to urinate in a cup, had to lay still for an EKG, and I had another chest x-ray snapped. I signed consent for surgery, got maps of the same hospital that I spent three years of my life in as a resident and knew well, and received pre-op instructions and special soap. No detail was overlooked.

After several hours, we had to go back to the radiology imaging site where I had my second CT in a week. Before this week, I had never even had a chest x-ray done! Here I was, IV in my arm again, iodine coursing in my veins, the warm sensation filling my chest, belly, and bladder as I stared at the Pac-Man faces, inhaling, holding my breath, exhaling, praying, "Let this be normal!" Afterwards, I had the privilege of having the radiologist look at the films with me on site. I saw images of my liver, my kidneys, my intestines, my adrenal glands, my uterus, and my bladder flash before me, but no other tumors! "Hallelujah" singing in my heart, I hugged my mom, and Shane and jumped up and down in victory! *I won't let this defeat me!* This long day was finally over. I felt lighthearted, somewhat relieved, and in a good mood. I would sleep better that night but certainly not the night before the big crack.

In a way, I already had felt like I had been cracked open. In the middle of being diagnosed with a tumor in my chest, I felt myself opening up and feeling more alive than ever. I started journaling and wanting to spend more time with God. Like I said, I wanted to deeply feel each moment—no denial, no pretending. This aliveness was strange and unexpected. A canyon was etched as the river of suffering and an unknown future washed over me. Apathy, ambivalence, doubt, and anxiety started flowing out of the crack of me. As my soul emptied, this left more room inside of me to be filled with other things. Spirit, calmness, and peace filtered into the crack. I was being filled with good, but I had to be cracked open for that to happen.

The night of May 25 I was on the phone with my most prayerful friends, curled up in a ball on my knees, my face in the pillow, crying, feeling my cup overflow as my friends blessed me over and over. Wanting to preserve the moment and remember what I looked like before surgery, I took pictures of my uncut, scalpel-free thorax. I wanted to feel strong for the next day, so I did some bicep curls and went for a run. I longed to feel God's presence, so I listened to praise music. Rest was important so I went to bed early, but I tossed and turned. I wanted to get the surgery over with. I wanted the devil out of me. I wanted to be cracked open, emptied of the bad, and filled with all things good. It was time.

May 26 was the day my chest was split wide open. The clock alarm went off at 4:00 a.m. that morning. By 4:05, I was in the shower trying to open my sticky eyes tired from nonsleep and worry. I scrubbed my skin with the unmistakable scent of chlorhexidine, the hospital-provided translucent pink liquid surgical soap. Knowing in less than four hours that the surgeon would use a scalpel and then a saw down the middle of my breastbone, I lathered up my chest several times. I guess I was hoping to wash away whatever was lurking underneath my scar-free skin! Naked, I stood in front of the large plate glass mirror in the bathroom with the glaring Hollywood lights, and I stared at my chest. I ran my index finger down the center and tried to imagine what I would look like tomorrow, wounded and stitched up. Since I wasn't allowed to eat, put on makeup, or even wear my wedding ring, it didn't take long to get ready. I dressed in black velour warm-up pants and a matching zip-front jacket. I was told not to wear anything I would have to pull over my head because I wouldn't be able to get it on or off after they were done with me! After I got dressed, I plugged in my new favorite CDs and fell to my knees on the living room floor, face in the carpet, arms open wide, touching the hem of heaven and praying for complete peace and hope that the elephant in my chest would be gone by tomorrow.

We were at the hospital and in the pre-op area by 4:45 that morning. Usually getting up that early in the morning is the hardest part of the day, but I am sure on this particular day my mom and husband would totally disagree. The worst for them was yet to come…

I, on the other hand, had reached a rare existential moment where I felt completely safe and secure. I was in God's hands. I literally felt like God was in me, and I was in God. I felt like what a small trickle of a cool creek water traveling hundreds of miles would feel when it drips into the huge ocean, and they become one and the same body. If something horrible was about to happen, I knew deep in my heart that heaven was where I would trickle next. I realized this was much easier for me to say than it was for my loved ones to hear. I knew that I had to keep my spirit alive, and that is where some of the most memorable, anesthesia-laced surgery stories were born.

The first of these stories started in the pre-op holding area when I was taken and separated from my family. I had on a non-one-of-a-kind blue hospital gown, and I lay underneath a pile of blankets trying to stay warm. I was transported on a gurney along the long hospital corridors to the sterile holding gut of the operating room. I was the first case of the day, so the hallways were still and quiet, like me. I was introduced to nurses and anesthesiologists and assistants and a chaplain. My arms were poked, and the lifeblood of my veins and arteries was accessed as the OR seemed to come to life. I think I was given something in my IV to remain calm but maybe not. I was grateful when my husband and my mom were brought to me one more time before the surgery started. I was called to go. The surgeon was ready. My family gave me hugs and kisses, and I told them that I would see them very soon—the surgery was only scheduled to last forty-five minutes— only forty-five minutes to crack me open, take out the mass, get a diagnosis, and put me back together! That would be a short forty-five minutes for me, and a long forty-five minutes for my family.

As I was being wheeled feet first into the mysterious depths of the surgical suite, I started to softly sing, "Shout to the Lord." I heard my family saying, "I love you!" I remember lifting my right arm up high in the air, giving them the thumbs-up sign, and I kept on singing, "Glory and majesty, praise to the King!" I felt someone touch my right arm and gently lower it back to the bedside. The nurse didn't want me to dislodge an IV or hit anyone on my way to the OR, I guess. My fighting spirit wouldn't have it. I raised my right arm up again, this time fast and even higher! "Mountains bow down and the seas will roar at the sound of Your name!" I sang. The transportation technician turned and looked at my husband and shrugged his shoulders. My husband smiled and did the same. That was the moment my husband said that he knew that I was going to be just fine.

The second most memorable event on the day that I was cracked open happened later in the morning after surgery. I awoke out of the deepest slumber. *Where was I? Home? Hotel? Oh, yeah, I was in the hospital!* My eyes felt like they were full of ointment, and my lashes were oily and thick. Everything looked blurry. *Was I awake?* I was trying to be! Someone was shaking my left shoulder. It was my surgeon. "Holly," I heard him say, "did they tell you yet?

I thought to myself, *Who are "they"? What were "they" supposed to tell me?*

"You have lymphoma," I heard him say next.

I knew it. I don't know how much time passed, but suddenly, and only for a brief second, I was aware that my husband and my mother were in the room. On pins and needles, afraid, yet curious of what my response was going to be, one of them asked me, "Did you understand what he just told you? You have lymphoma."

My eyes were sleepy, oily, blurry. *Why can't I wake up all the way? I have to talk to them. Let me just say this one thing!* And out of my groggy lips, bubbling up from my spirit within, I heard myself say, "I hate it when I'm right!" My surgeon and my family laughed. And that was when my mother knew that I was going to be just fine.

People say that things come in threes, and sure enough, there was a third event that I recall with uncanny clarity on the day that I was cracked open. In and out of my anesthetized brain and floating on the breeze of some pretty strong pain medications, I don't remember most of that blurry first day in the intensive care unit. What I do remember is that every time I woke up, I couldn't see a thing! I am one of those people who is heavily dependent on contact lenses or a pair of glasses—I can't see without them! I guess I slept a lot that first day, and the hospital day shift came and went. I woke up in the middle of the night. I heard weird gurgling noises, and for the first time, I realized that the noises were coming from me and my chest tubes! I, healthy me, had chest tubes in my body! *Oh, yeah, I have cancer. I have to rest. I wonder what time it is.* I looked at the clock that was up high on the wall in front of me. I squinted trying to read the hands. *Four o'clock in the morning! Victory! Only three more hours until the next shift change! That means I made it through the first twenty-four hours since the surgery. Soon I can get these noisy chest tubes out of me. And, oh man, I probably have a catheter in too. That's gotta go! Get me out of the ICU and into a normal room!* I called out to my nurse, and he came. "What can I do for you?" he politely asked.

"Nurse," I said, "what time is it? Is it 4:00 in the morning?"

He smiled at me. "No. Dr. Johnson, it is 10:00 at night."

Dang it! I laughed to myself. *This is nuts! I have a long way to go until 7:00 shift change. I must be cracking up to think it was 4:00 in the morning! I need to sleep off some more of these pain meds!*

The next day finally did arrive, and the medical team did pull out my chest tubes, one in each side. *I don't want to have that ever again!* They pulled out the catheter. They pulled out some IVs and left one. I got out of the ICU. They gave me my glasses! I was there for four more days until I could walk a lap around the hallways and until I could poop. They make a big deal about poop before you can go home. Then, after five of the longest days of my life, I went home to recover.

Project: Tumor Annihilation and Mission: Remission

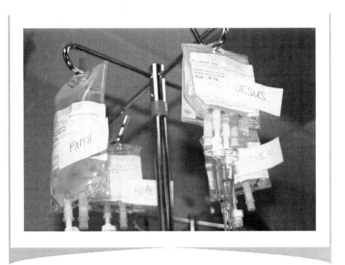

Photo by the author

The day I renamed my chemo meds:
Jesus, Faith, Hope, and Love.

RX: Find your mojo. Get a tattoo. Have a ritual.

Six days after my surgery, I finally felt well enough to get out of the house and travel past my front yard. My mom, my brother, Eric, and I drove to Park Avenue in Winter Park, Florida. This is a quaint street lined with boutique stores, eateries, and rose gardens. We slipped down a side street, a frozen yogurt store beckoning to us. It was hot outside. The taste of cool treat on our tongues would soothe us all. As we walked into the store, I saw retro minichandeliers made of white-and-black plastic small circles hanging from the ceiling. Throwback, plastic, white barrel chairs were scattered across the concrete floor and a high-backed black suede couch lined one wall. I sat on the couch by myself while Mom and Eric stood in line. It was quiet and thoughts of a yogurt swirl were getting to my head. First, my eyes got watery. Then, before I knew it, I was weeping uncontrollably. Suddenly the fear of the unknown, and the knowledge of what was surely coming, all hit me and blew me down like a dandelion in the wind.

> I am a cancer patient; this week I will undergo many tests, and I will start chemotherapy. My oncologist will become my lifeboat. A new reality is slipping into my life. The medications will attack the tumor, and I will take other medications to help prevent nausea. But what if it doesn't work? What if the tumor doesn't go away?

My mom and Eric brought me a cup of yogurt, I took a bite, and I hated the taste of it. I started crying even harder then. I couldn't stop. We had to leave and go home.

Two days later, I woke up in the dark, and Shane and my mom took me to my first PET scan. This scan would allow the doctor to tell me the stage of my cancer. The lower the number, the lower the stage, the better. At the nuclear medicine imaging center, I checked in, paid my $200 co-pay, and I was led to a room with a gray, lazy-boy chair. I hopped into the chair and started shivering. The tech brought me some institutionalized off-white-colored, scratchy, but warm blankets and explained the PET scan procedure. An IV was started in my arm, and I was handed a Styrofoam cup of vanilla-lemon-flavored contrast to drink. *Who dreamed up that flavor combination?* I wondered. My mom wanted to taste it, too, so she stuck her tongue in the cup and then made a face. I gulped the rest of it down and chased it with a bottle of water. The tech brought in a silver thermos with a side arm and cock stop with a syringe attached to it. This was the super-radioactive nuclear medicine contrast that in another two seconds would be infused into my veins, which don't have any insulation like the thermos! *Holy cow, that can't be inhaled by human lungs or touched by human hands, but it has to run though me?!?* I got a little nervous. The mysterious liquid was drawn into the syringe and then attached to the IV in my arm. In it went—I felt the coolness of the infusion sneak up into my arm. Then I was given another Styrofoam cup of vanilla-lemon joy to gulp down, and I was told to shut my eyes and to not talk for the next hour.

An hour later, they came to get me as promised, and I was led to the PET scan room. The machine looked like an MRI machine with a table that slid into a narrow tube. I lay down, they covered me with blankets, and they told me that they would be done in twenty-two minutes. I closed my eyes. I felt the table rise, and I was slid into the tube of the PET scanner. I felt the blankets bunch up around my shoulders. I sang praise songs inside my head, being careful not to let my lips move or my toes twitch to the music that I imagined that I was hearing. When there was one minute to go, the tech let me know. Excited to be almost done, I allowed my eyes to flutter open, just for a brief moment, and I was shocked to see that the inner part of the machine was only about an inch and a half from the tip of my nose. I panicked! I was not expecting that! I didn't like it one bit! Anxiety rolled over me like another blanket, and suddenly, I was hot, and I wanted out! Somehow, I calmed myself, and I remained still for the last sixty seconds in PET scan hell. *I need a Xanax.*

Later in the day, my oncologist called me at home. It was good news. The only hot spot on the scan was the tumor itself and some small surrounding lymph nodes. No other organs or bone marrow were involved! I was so excited to be stage IIA and not stage III or IV! He told me to plan to have six rounds (or twelve treatments) of chemotherapy every other week (well, maybe four rounds) and then four weeks of radiation. He asked me how I was doing, and I told him about my breakdown on Park Avenue. These are the healing words that he said back to me,

You will be the same person you are in one month, two months, six months as you are today. You will live just as long into the future with or without this disease. Nothing will disable you. You are healthy. You will fit these treatments into your life, and these treatments will not dominate your life. You didn't deserve this. There are many people in your life, patients included, who need you. You are in control. God is in control.

His words empowered me. I was still me. God was (and is) in control. I wanted to follow His will and to do what I do best: get organized and pep myself up! In this moment I realized that no one was going to do this for me. People in my life started to tell me how strong I am. The truth was that I did not feel strong at all; I just refused to fall apart. This wasn't a time to be strong and pretend that everything was all right. This was a time for me to find joy wherever I could.

To chase joy and to get my cancer organized, first I claimed the moment and I named it—Project: Tumor Annihilation, and when that was accomplished, other projects followed. There would be Mission: Remission, and then finally, Mission: Cure I decided! I ran to my favorite Target store and bought notebooks, dividers, three ring binders, highlighters; and I went to work. I highly recommend a burst of organizational energy for anyone going through a crisis that leaves a trail of paperwork and fills your mind with an endless source of questions. In my binder, there were tabs for labs, x-rays, bills, hospital information, and cancer facts; and in my handheld notebook, there were sections for vital signs and my weight, the most important labs like my white blood cell count and hemoglobin, a cancer "to do" list, and questions to ask my different doctors. The notebooks filled up fast, and I was grateful to have my health information all in one place early on and easily accessible. When I had "chemo brain" and my own head couldn't think fast enough, my peripheral brain (in my notebooks) helped me out immensely to recall facts and information.

Although I like to be prepared and for everything to be in its place, organizing my thoughts in three ring binders and page dividers wasn't really a joyful exercise, so I came up with a Mission: Remission ritual as well. Every night before a chemo treatment became my creative meditation time. First, I chose a temporary tattoo design from my collection. (The collection came from my brother who mailed me about fifty tattoos to use for my treatments. I told him, "What am I going to do with all of these?!? I only have twelve treatments, not fifty!" He assured me, "Don't worry. You will make friends!") I chose a tattoo design based on what made me happy in the moment, and I sat at the dining room table and meditated on the design for several minutes. I got out a piece of blank white paper and a black and a red marker. Then, by freehand, I drew my interpretation of the tattoo in the middle of the paper. Then at the top of the paper, I scrolled, "Project: Tumor Annihilation." Underneath my drawing, I wrote in big bold letters, "Round # 1," and under that I wrote, "Job 23:10 'I shall come forth as gold.'" I also decorated the corners of the paper with artistic curves and biker chic motifs. As I drew, I listened to music—the same three songs repeatedly until I was lulled to the bedroom to meditate in the quiet and put myself to sleep. (See the chapter called "Pick It and Flick It" for more about meditation.)

In the morning, I showered, put on my new tattoo above the right side of my chest, and in my family room, posed for the camera holding my hand-drawn sign, the morning light streaming through the windows. I packed up my notebooks, water bottle, blanket, iPod, and extra tattoos, and off I went in search of my own healing and new members of the chemo posse who might also like to start a Mission: Remission ritual.

My Chemo Posse

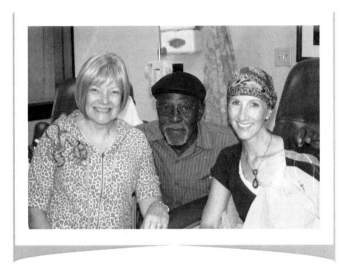

Photo by Shane Johnson

MaryAnne, Zeddy, and me. My faithful
partners in crime to beat up cancer.

RX: Make new friends. Often they will know just
what your heart needs before you even know.

I learned rather quickly even before starting treatment that cancer and other hard times in life do not understand boundaries, play favorites, or choose only certain character profiles. Here I was, thirty-nine years old, one of the healthiest people I knew, in the prime of my career with no family history of cancer and no other risks for developing cancer, and I was hit from the blindside with my new diagnosis. I knew that I didn't want to take on this monster alone. I needed people who understood on a heart level what I was thinking, feeling, and experiencing without me ever having to say a word. I was surprised how easily this came to me.

I met the president of my chemo posse in a chemotherapy class that I had to attend. In class, I sat next to a woman named MaryAnne who had silver-blond hair and bright blue eyes, which danced with delight whenever she would smile. When she smiled and laughed, joy took over her face, and her eyes squinted in merriment. She didn't look sick, and I wondered if she was even a patient or if she was just there supporting a loved one.

All the patients in the room were handed a purple folder with information about our diagnosis, the names and potential side effects of all of our medications, and when to call the physician's office. When a purple folder was handed to her, I knew that she was indeed a patient. What I didn't know was that she would become the leader of my posse! As our oncology nurse explained to us how our treatment days would go and overwhelmed us with information relevant to all of us, many of the patients and family members who gathered around the executive-sized table looked scared, nervous, sad, and intense. The woman next to me, however, listened intently and laughed along with me at the nurse's attempts at a few jokes. The nurse, for example, commented that most of us would lose our hair due to our treatment, but that it would grow back. She said, "It may come back straight or curly, but if it comes back gray, we won't take responsibility for that!" I chuckled and turned to the calm, composed lady next to me who cracked up; her laugh was infectious, and I joined in. I knew I had found a friend.

At the end of the class, I leaned over to her and said, "I don't know anything about you, but I love the warm energy that radiates from you. I have a deep sense, that whatever is wrong, you will be okay." She seemed unfazed by my comment and simply asked me about me. We figured out that we would be on the same chemo cycle and that we absolutely would see each other again. I was thrilled to have met my best chemo buddy. Without a word passing between us, MaryAnne already knew me from my inside place of fear, surgery scars, anxiety and wonder of chemotherapy and hair loss, and an unknown future. She became a fixture in my life in the weeks, months, and years ahead. She was such a thoughtful president of the club: if I was running late on a chemo day, she would put her big brown bag on the chair next to her and would save my seat until I got there! She also baked and brought homemade health-conscious treats and lugged boxes of popsicles in a cooler to our treatments and shared with everyone. She amazed me!

One time, the week of our second dose of medications, I walked to the chair she had saved for me next to a fish tank housing a big orange fish with big lips. She met me with her huge grin, reached to the back of her head, pulled out a clump of her short blond hair, and said, "Look! I'm going to shave my head this week!" I couldn't believe it—she looked ecstatic about this new baldness adventure! She was showing me maturity and humor in one bite. I took the bait, and I was bolstered for my eventual turn with the inevitable.

After I had my first hair cut, I went to visit her in her beautiful Mediterranean-mission-style house, and she opened the door with a blond wig on. I had never seen her with a wig on, and that was the first time she had seen my short, pixie-style cut. When she saw me, she put her hands to her face and screeched, "Look at your hair!"

I screeched back, "Look at your hair! You got your wig! You look amazing!" Then I asked, "Is it hot under there, and does it itch at all?"

MaryAnne, ever the crusader, put her right hand high over her head, where it lit on top of her, and she plucked that head of hair right off her bald scalp, and said, "Here! You try!" Howling with laughter, it took several minutes before we could speak another word to each other.

There was strength in knowing I wasn't going at this alone. Thinking of MaryAnne and other members of my posse was like having an extra biceps muscle I could flex at any time and lift any load that was put in front of me. MaryAnne and other patients became my inspiration to spread as much encouragement during our time together that I could. I shared music on my iPod with other patients, wrote some of them notes of encouragement, and spent time just listening to their hopes and dreams. The pendulum swung both ways. Times when I felt discouraged and weak, and I didn't feel like facing another treatment, I would be at home grudgingly preparing to ride to the hospital, and I would think to myself, I have to go, MaryAnne and the posse will be there saving my seat! This story of mine would be very different if it weren't for this special clan—this mosaic of personalities woven into my chemo days.

MaryAnne and I did our best to recruit other members of the posse. One was a thin, seventy-something-year-old, black man named Zeddy who would come plop himself down in one of the lazy-boy chemo chairs on either side of us, hat turned slightly sideways, grinning, his poor dentition flashing at us. He was a sarcastic fellow and delighted us with his grumpiness and flirtatious manner with the nurses. One time I asked him if he had trouble sleeping at night after his treatments like I did. He said, "No, not really. If I wake up, I jist roll over, grab a snack, roll back over, chew, and go back ta sleep."

I asked him, "Zeddy, what is your favorite thing to eat in the middle of the night?"

He unabashedly answered, "Either Oreos or potato chips. Don't ask me to pick a favorite! I like 'em both!"

I said, "Zeddy, you're going to lose some teeth eating that way in the middle of the night!"

His reply was something along the lines of, "Mizz Holly, I don't have eyelashes anymore; ya think I care 'bout the few teeth I have left?"

This seventy-year-old, who looked like he was fifty, was more concerned about having some hair on his head for his son's upcoming wedding than he was about his teeth rotting out from his midnight snacks! As you can imagine, he slipped into our chemo posse without a hitch and called us "His Women."

There was another young girl that I spotted one day after I had already been through a couple of treatments. Her doting mother accompanied her. She sat slumped in her chair, head in her hands, fear in her eyes. She was a quieter member of the posse, and it took a few weeks before she felt comfortable sharing her story. Her name was Karen (and we have the same birthday, exactly one year apart)! She loved the outdoors, was a runner, and a nurse. She signed all her e-mails to me with an "XOXO." She was a married woman with two boys. Her family was moving to the Bahamas, and they had stopped in Orlando to see friends when she developed flu-like symptoms and went to the emergency room where physicians didn't find the flu—they found metastatic kidney cancer. Watching Karen go through her treatments was the first time I had ever watched a friend week by week dying in front of me. At first, she became thin. Her bones started to hurt. Then, as her cancer ate her from the inside out, she became swollen, and she lost the light in her blue-green eyes.

She told me, "Holly, I'm so scared!" I bought her the softest slippers I could find for her swollen feet for our birthday. She died within six months of becoming a member of the posse. Losing her felt like a punch in the stomach; it felt like losing a game to a cheating player named Cancer. It was haunting. It was not fair, and I know what the rest of the posse all thought, *That could have been me.*

Mrs. Bradley was another member of the club. She was in her eighties with silver-white hair brushed off her wide forehead, big brown eyes, and big eyeglasses. She wore large square house dresses that rivaled my grandma's. Her thick ankles swelled out from under her dresses. She didn't actually have cancer; she had anemia of chronic disease, which meant her blood counts were always low, and there wasn't a reason for it, but she had to have iron infusions to keep her alive. She was often tired and short of breath, yet she had an air of regality about her. MaryAnne and I introduced ourselves one day, and we found out she and her husband were part of the long history of Florida Hospital. He was an administrator, and she was a nurse. She delighted us with stories about the hospital's early days when it was nothing but a house on a lake in the middle of cow pasture. Her husband was still the keeper of an early recording book that had the names of surgical patients in the front of the ledger and the number of gallons of milk each Florida Hospital cow produced in the back of the ledger! One day, Mrs. Bradley looked so sad as she sat in her chair. She started to cry. I floated over to her and told her I had something for her. She looked at me with curiosity, and as I leaned over her, I put my arms around her and gave her a hug. I said the same words my pastor had said to me at my anointing, "God has you." Ever since that day, the two of us have passed Bible verses back and forth to one another in encouragement. She was the spiritual ambassador of the group.

The posse was a special place, and anyone who sat in a chair in the back of the oncologist's office knew it well. The posse grew and shrank from session to session as some finished treatments and others passed on to a different phase. Just like invasive cancer cells did not discriminate, the posse didn't either. There were patients with breast cancer, lung cancer, Kaposi's sarcoma, stomach and esophageal cancer, and blood disorders. We were young and old, black and white, and living and dying, but it only took one look from the outside to see that something special was going on inside of the posse. We were women and men huddled close, like a tribal council around a bursting campfire. We protected one another, kept the fire burning, and promised that no one would ever get voted off our island!

One Out of Twelve

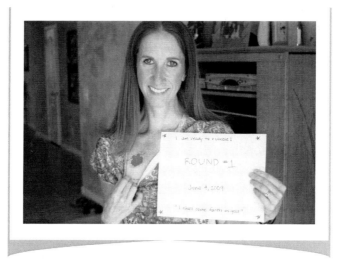

Photo by Shane Johnson

Ready to rumble before my first chemo treatment.

RX: Listen to your doctors.

June 4 was my first day of chemotherapy. I woke up with calmness in my soul and complete trust in the Lord and my treatment plan. I took one of the longest showers I can ever remember, relishing the feel of my long hair, shampooing and conditioning each strand. *Since I am having chemo today, will I be bald tomorrow or next week? How long will it take for my hair to fall out?* I hadn't even lost any hair yet, and I was asking myself, *how long will it take for it all to grow back?* After my indulgent shower, I placed a temporary tattoo on the right side of my upper chest: a red heart floating on a bed of red roses with fine background detail of black outlined modern, funky triangles. A new tattoo every other week became my mojo, a metaphoric energy that I changed every two weeks to bring myself joy and bring a smile to my chemotherapy nurses.

The ride to the hospital was long. My mother drove (I still wasn't allowed behind the wheel due to my big crack!) and my husband met us there. "There" is the Cancer Institute at Florida Hospital, suite 286, where I would entrust my life and future in four chemotherapy medications—ABVD: adriamycin, bleomycin, vincristine, and dacarbazine, which my mother lovingly dubbed apples, bananas, violets, and daisies so she could remember them better. When I arrived at my first appointment, Linda, Dr. Reynolds' nurse, took out the sutures where my chest tubes had been. I was greeted by Dr. Reynolds and introduced to many of the staff. I walked into the back of the office, which had a big L-shaped area of brown leather lazy-boy type chairs that surrounded a nurses' station. I chose a chair near the corner of the L where I could see people coming and going, my haptic awareness point for the next five hours, and most importantly, it was near the bathroom!

I saw my new friend, MaryAnne, whom I met in the chemo class. (She is the woman with short, silver-blond hair, bright blue eyes, who had the positive vibe radiating all around her.) We were on the same chemo cycle, and I was sure that I would learn more about her as the days and months of treatment went on.

Once I sat in my chair of choice, and after a few nervous bathroom breaks, my treatment day was explained, and my nurse was chosen for me. Her name was Katina. She was every bit of what an angel will look like in heaven someday. She was younger than me, larger than me, and darker than me. She had deep milk-chocolate skin and a brilliant smile of big gappy teeth. Her hair was short and spiky. She loved my tattoo and showed me hers. Hers was permanent. On the back of her left shoulder was the outline of the back of an angel with blue wings and a halo. Katina looked at me in the eye when she spoke to me, her hands were warm, and I trusted her immediately.

To get the medicines inside of me every other week, I had something called a port surgically sewn into my upper left chest. This port was called a "Power Port," and it was a little purple plastic triangle with a rubber ball in the center and a long tail that went into one of my veins. I could easily see and feel my port, a "third nipple" on my surgically scarred chest. Katina just had to feel for the rubber ball and poke into it with a special needle. Then the healing juices could flow! As my port was accessed for the first time, it was a painful poke in my tender and still-swollen chest.

Once at peace and filled with the spirit, I suddenly lost control, fear crept in, and I wept as reality slapped me from the left and right. I had cancer, and this was my new reality. I wasn't living a dream or someone else's life. This was about me, and I was about to be treated for cancer. *This is deep and serious, and I am scared.* I was comforted by the laying on of hands and voices of many including my mom, Shane, and several nurses. One of the other patients saw my tearful face, and she came over to me, patted my hand, and relayed a story to me about someone young and beautiful that she met on her first chemo day. This young and beautiful patient had a very positive outlook and that strength in her was passed on to this other woman who was now passing it on to me. She asked about my diagnosis, and when I told her that I had Hodgkin's lymphoma, she quickly smiled, pulled her shoulders back, and with conviction exclaimed, "That is great news! That is highly curable!" Caught off guard by her confidence and enthusiasm, I thought to myself, *I love those words, and I will live that out!* I am telling you, there is strength in numbers. I was soon able to regroup and focus on my healing once again.

Once my port was accessed, I was given an intravenous antinausea medication and steroids, then my first dose of vincristine. While that was infusing, the nurse came over to me to place a test dose of bleomycin underneath the skin of my left forearm. Katina told me, "This will just feel like you are getting a test for tuberculosis." I thought to myself, *No big deal*. I can handle a TB test. That is a cakewalk compared to her poking my chest to get into the port and compared to having open chest surgery! Well, I was very wrong about that! That test dose burned and stung and hurt me more than anything else I had felt in weeks! It ended up blistering my skin, and I have a scar to this day from that test dose of bleomycin. I thought, *If that is what it does to my skin, it better be in there destroying this lymphoma!* Once the test dose was done, and the vincristine was done, the adriamycin was started—bright-red juice flowing into me. This was the magic potion that would make my hair fall out and make my urine turn red! Many people call it "The Red Devil," but Katina and I called it my "Jesus Juice." As the adriamycin dripped from the IV bag, I stared at it as it flowed into the IV line, directly into my power port, and into my body. I imagined it fighting for me. (Within a half hour, at my next bathroom break, I peeked in the toilet. Sure enough, red, peachy-colored pee! I thought that was hilarious and awesome and couldn't wait to pull up my pants—without getting tangled in my web of IVs—and go tell my husband and text my brother!) Then the third medication, the bleomycin was given, and lastly, the dacarbazine. My mom and Shane sat across from me patiently watching, waiting, reading, meditating as they witnessed the start of my cure. I read a little, listened to music, prayed, and slept. Dr. Reynolds stopped by a few times to check in on me. He told me that my tumor was a stage IIA. That meant I was automatically signed up for six months of chemotherapy, every other week, for twelve total treatments, followed by four weeks of radiation treatment.

When I finished my first round of twelve chemotherapy treatments, I was able to get up and walk away feeling okay. Tired, but okay, knowing I could now go home! I was starving, so I wolfed down a turkey sandwich! I couldn't believe how good it tasted! I then sent some e-mails and rested and relaxed. Dinner was steak on the grill, which also tasted really good! I was so thankful for a great appetite and no nausea or vomiting like most of the cancer stories in movies and books portray.

The next day, I faced my day-after-chemo-treatment day. I had to go back to the cancer center, get my port accessed again, and receive intravenous fluids, more antinausea medication, and a shot in my arm called Neulasta. This shot boosted my white blood cell count to protect me from infections and to keep me healthy. Then I would do this cycle all over again in two weeks. Chemo Thursdays and Neulasta Fridays. Never have I wished that time could go so slow and so fast at the same time.

Love in a Biscuit

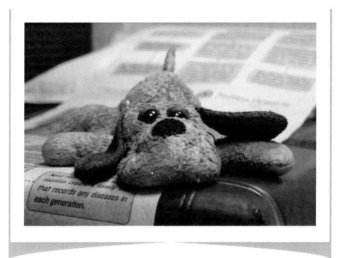

Photo by the author

My favorite get-well gift: Biscuit.

RX: Believe in love like a five-year-old. Your boo-boos will get better.

I was overwhelmed with the response of friends and family members who stepped forward and took time out of their days to send me a letter, flowers, or cookies, type me an e-mail, or call on the phone when they heard that I was gearing up for the fight of my life. I literally have a twelve-inch-by-twelve-inch-by-twelve-inch box chock-full of get-well cards and sentiments that were sent to me...and I will keep them forever. They connected me with each loved one on a heart level, and they still bring me to tears of joy when I reread them. Some of these cards sang to me, some made me think, some made me cry, and all made me grateful. Many of my friends had their kids sit down at their kitchen tables and draw me pictures and write some words to me. These are adorable construction paper artworks with random stick figures and streaks of big, fat crayon. Then, the paper was often folded, but not quite perfectly, into a card-sized packet or creative origami and presented to me with a big, fat hug. I loved getting these special treats, but seriously, it was often overwhelming. I didn't realize how many friends I really had or how many lives I was intertwined with. I was on prayer chains all over the United States (and Ghana!). Getting cancer was truly an *It's a Wonderful Life* moment for me.

One of the best gifts that I received was a carefully thought out get-well package from friends who work with my husband: all counselors in a middle school. The package was a bag of goodies and each little piece was wrapped and had a special note on it, encouraging me to get well and to use the contents to aid in my healing. With anticipation and curiosity overriding my fatigue for the moment, I remember sitting on the couch after one of my Neulasta Fridays, and I unwrapped the gifts one by one, relishing in the meaning of each treasure. Here is what I found: first, there was a dark raspberry-red journal with a magnetic clasp closure. The advice that came with the journal stated that it was a special journal and that I should use as I went though the healing process. "It's a counselor thing!" the note said. Those blank pages in that leather-bound portfolio were the very ones that I used to start writing this book. Through chronicling my days, my thoughts, my feelings, what I ate, and when I took my medications, I found that the feel of a pencil in my hand and watching words come to life on those pages did make me feel better and did help me in the healing process.

From the care package, I also found an incredibly soft, light-gray-colored blanket to use in case I needed to stay warm during my chemotherapy treatments. I didn't know that indeed I would get cold while sitting still for four to five hours at a time while I was being infused, so the blanket came with me to each treatment. Also in the goody bag was an orange insulated travel mug to tote green tea or other warm beverage in it. Sprawled across the mug in big white letters it said, "Momma told me there be days like this!" (Well, my momma certainly didn't expect the day would come when her daughter had cancer, but she sure taught me that there would be rough, unexpected days!) One of the most fun gadgets in the get-well package was an "Easy Button" that was bright orange, and when you pushed it, it sang "I Will Survive" by Debbie Harry. I was told to "use as necessary" and use it to remind myself that I would get through this; I will beat this! I will survive! I unwrapped chocolates, an iTunes gift card, and an adorable notepad with a yellow lab puppy sitting on a chair with its little head cocked at the camera.

There was the book, *Twilight*, with a note attached saying, "Welcome to middle school—stay young at heart with some girl drama." I thought I would never start reading this teeny-bopper series, but now I found that I had all the time in the world to dedicate myself to the addicting world of werewolves and vampires. I found healing in the escape to another world of Bella, Edward, and Jacob. I could forget about myself for hours reading thousands of pages in this series! Like these three characters, I was also undergoing a sort of transformation. My own body was staging a revolution so that I could undergo an evolution. Losing myself in these books was intentional healing for me! The introduction to the teenage vampire world, however, wasn't the best part of that care package.

The last token in the care package was a gift that became a symbol of love. Placed carefully on top of a stack of books in a bag of its own was a stuffed animal—a little dog named Biscuit. He was a well-worn in (or worn out!) caramel-colored, pill-balled, gnarly little furball. His ears were a darker brown color and very floppy. He had big brown, sad-looking, crooked, plastic glossy crossed eyes, and a tiny tail. The stuffing in Biscuit was distributed mostly in his head and back side. A collar of straw raffia decorated his skinny rag doll neck. The note attached to Biscuit said, "Holly, I know he is not the newest doggy, but my five-year-old wanted you to have Biscuit, his lovey from when he was a baby and who always made his boo-boos better."

Later I would learn that my friend was using my trial of lifetime as a teachable moment for her son, Griffin. She wanted to pull more empathy and compassion out of him. She came home from work the day that she found out that I was going to have surgery and told her son about my situation. She told him that she was going to make a care package for me, and she wanted to know if there was anything he wanted to put in the package. He went into his room for several minutes. He was very quiet. My friend was patient and went about preparing dinner and cleaning up around the house. When he finally came out, he handed Biscuit to my friend and said, "When I don't feel good, Biscuit always makes me feel better, so maybe he will help Mrs. Johnson to feel better too! Let's put him in the package!" That's not the end. The story gets even better...

The love that I found pouring out of that five-year-old was now woven into the threads that held Biscuit together. Biscuit, and therefore love, went with me to every treatment and PET scan, and I perched him on the footboard of the bed to watch over me at night. I held on to love, empathy, and compassion for the duration of my treatment. Eventually, when I did get better and my boo-boo was fixed, I knew that Biscuit needed to go home to Griffin. When this little boy found out that Biscuit was coming home to him, he was thrilled and so excited to be getting his favorite stuffed animal back! But after the excitement passed and he understood that I was healed, Griffin surprised us again. He said, "Mom, maybe Mrs. Johnson should keep him so that she never gets sick again!"

Love comes in many forms and rarely is it unconditional. For me, it came the year I had cancer. It came in a Biscuit.

High Tide

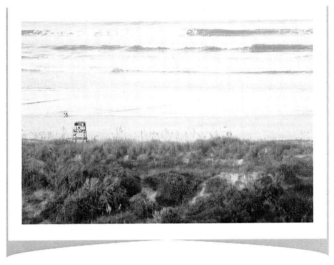

Photo by the author

New Smyrna Beach at sunrise during
a weekend with friends.

RX: Rise up. Move out of the mess, out of the debris.

We are born out of it. We drink it to live. We use it to wash our wounds and grow our grass. Over 90 percent of the earth is covered with it. Sixty percent of a human body is made of it. It forms our tears and cools our skin. We are baptized in it. It cools us off; it warms us up. It is a sustainer of life; it is life. It is water…It is my retreat.

The weekend before my surgery, then less than two weeks afterwards, and every vacation, every retreat I could take, I was called to the water. I wanted, more than anything, to stand at the brink of liquid and solid, to stare off at the horizon, and to contemplate our ancestors' thought that the earth must be flat. What is beyond what we cannot see in this world and inside of me?

I love to sit and stare at the waves chasing each other to shore, foaming at the mouth, then retreating; and when there is time before the next wave hits, I watch the rim of water seemingly melt into the sand. I marvel at how much noise just water alone can make as this process is repeated thousands of times throughout the day.

I also love to stand close to the edge of where the waves hit the beach—where the leftover foam looks like root beer—and let the water swirl around my skinny ankles. Then, as the water retreats back to where it came from, my feet feel like they are standing on platform shoes made out of wet sand. Eventually my feet are buried in it. I become a part of the sea. I am thrilled with this idea, and I believe that I should always stay here—at the beach, that is.

Walking for miles and watching the endless stretches of sand and people who are here to do the same thing as me—retreat, relax, refresh—connects me to the planet. I bend over to inspect a purple moon shell or other treasure that the sea has coughed up—beads, plastic army figures, sand dollars, and pink beach shovels. I pocket and save them all. I wonder, how far did this have to travel to land at my feet, at the seam of earth and water?

The beach is an impressive metaphor for life. Sometimes it is as calm and gentle as a mother's hand stroking her baby's head; other times, it rages from the depths and tosses around the most indestructible ship there is. Water can appear so harmless on the outside, but then the invisible riptides, the under-the-surface sea creatures, and the fast-approaching storms can really surprise us and hurt. Ahhhh, the ocean—so wide, so vast, so blue—always speaking to us as the sounds of the water crest and fall. Sometimes the waves crash to the sand, and sometimes they whisper, leaving little gifts of shells and sea glass: gifts we can palm in our hands and feel the heartbeat of the ocean beckoning us to stay or at least to come back soon. With that promise, it brings a new tide, a promise of a new day as the sun rises out of it on the east coast and leaves us breathless as it sinks into the water kissing us good night on the west coast.

Ocean, lake, river, stream, it doesn't matter to the soul. The soul knows water. It knows the need for baptism: worries can be washed away and hurts can be left behind. The soul understands that water replenishes life and brings life to our senses. Water washes us clean, but first, we must get in it. When we are faced with the enemy, I believe we can count on the sea to bring us back to our senses and ground us even more. Thank you, Hilton Head, New Smyrna Beach, Diamond Lake, shores of Ka'anapali, Bar Harbor, and Long Lake. During the days I felt like I was drowning, you instead pulled me in, renewed my soul, and spit me back out. When I visit you, I can, like a wet dog, shake off my days—cancer, misery, and pain seem to spiral off me—and again I can come up for air.

Barbara Kingsolver says it best in her book *High Tide in Tuscon*,

> Every one of us is called upon, probably many times, to start a new life. A frightening diagnosis, a marriage, a move, a loss of a job...And onward full tilt we go, pitched and wrecked and absurdly resolute, driven in spite of everything to make good on a new shore. To be hopeful, to embrace one possibility after another —that is surely the basic instinct... Crying out: High Tide! Time to move out into the glorious debris. Time to take this life for what it is!

Pick It and Flick It

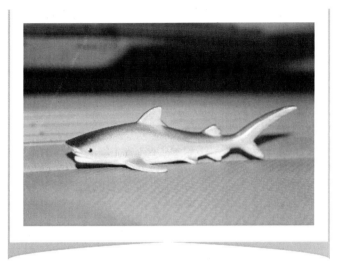

Photo by the author

Sharky, the tumor chomping ninja!

RX: Meditate.

My husband and I love to travel. Between the two of us, we have been to forty-seven states, twenty countries, and four continents. The world is our oyster when we travel. We love to meet new people. We love to see as many mountains, rivers, college campuses, sports arenas, national parks, and wildlife we can possibly see in a lifetime. We love blending with other cultures and hearing other languages. When we travel, we collect ornaments for our Christmas tree and often pick up other souvenirs along the way.

One hot summer, we were in Niagara Falls, Canada, when a special token came our way. It was free of charge, found laying in a parking lot, probably accidentally fallen from a kiddy backpack when Mom was stuffing her family back into an SUV to drive to the next vacation destination. My husband and I had finished eating our Grand Slam breakfast at Denny's and walked out into the parking area. As I opened the passenger door to the red Kia Rio rental car, my husband hurled something over the roof toward me! I ducked, thinking he was trying to spook me with a big spider or something else boyish and gross.

It landed at my feet. A two-inch souvenir, plastic, gray-colored great white shark, dorsal fin and all, stared up at me from the pavement. I mimicked a scream, "Shark!" I picked him up, sat down in the toasty car seat, and put "Sharky" on the dashboard. That shark not only drove all over Canada with us, it also came home with us and now travels in my white Honda Fit wherever I go. And when it is time to go on a trip away from home, somehow it magically makes its way to the dashboard of our latest rental car.

Sharky became a symbol of safety and security. It is our mobile dashboard ornament guiding us through traffic, zipping on and off the interstates, and accompanying us on our journeys. Little did I know, many years after Sharky joined us in Niagara, this little plastic creature would become a huge part of my road to recovery.

Many counselors and spiritual mentors recommend using guided imagery to their clients who are facing chronic diseases, addictions, and cancer. The theory is that the mind-body-spirit connection is so strong that when practiced regularly, a strong mental image of something or someone fighting a crisis and winning that crisis will actually come to fruition in the physical form. When you think positive thoughts long enough and hard enough, your body thinks that these thoughts are real and also reacts in a positive way. If you make your thoughts real enough and actively guide images in your brain to heal you, the body simply follows. My counselor says that as we use imagery, our bodies don't know what is not real. Our bodies, our cells, our living inner being actually believe that this imagery is really happening.

Fighting for my life, healing from surgery, under-going chemotherapy, and taking some medications proactively to prevent some symptoms and some reactively to stop pain, I was compelled not only to do whatever my doctors told me to do but also to pray and meditate. After all, there are no side effects to prayer and meditation! I knew I wanted to meditate my tumor away, but I had no idea what image to use. Not to be discouraged, I remembered reading somewhere that often the meditator doesn't find the image but rather the image finds the meditator.

Determined to start my own meditation ritual, I lay back in my bed on top of the chocolate-brown sheets and a couple of pillows, and I closed my eyes. "This bed is your tumor annihilator," my husband said. I imagined the tumor in my chest, nestled in the dark space between my heart and lungs, my pulmonary vessels, and my bronchial tubes. I imagined it was light tan and the texture of a soft, gritty pear. I imagined that it was on a short stalk, oval shaped, freely floating inside a sea of salty protoplasm. As I conjured up this very vivid picture, guess what swam around the corner of my right ventricle and took a chomp out of my lymphoma? It was Sharky! A symbol of safety, security, and surely strength, that little plastic fearless token found its way into the fish tank of my chest and started eating my tumor! I could see its jaws lurch forward. There were rows of triangular, sharp teeth gnashing and tearing away at the tumor. It swam around, scanning for the best attack angle, chomping the tumor, and avoiding the healthy stuff like my blood vessels and nerves. It ate until it could eat no more.

I meditated like that for ten to fifteen minutes every day. I believed in Sharky so much that after several weeks, meditation became easy for me. I looked forward to this quiet time of prayer and complete concentration on the edibility of my cancer. Over time, I visualized my tumor getting smaller. With a shrinking tumor, Sharky started to become hesitant to chomp and gnaw for fear of injuring me and my vital organs. *Now what was I going to do?* My mind could still see free floating clumps of cancer cells, and Sharky was no longer going for the bait.

The next day, I was curious and anxious as I lay down to pray and use my personal guided imagery. I closed my eyes. The fish tank inside my chest filled with a murky water, and I saw my great white hero swimming in and out of the foreground. Suddenly, a different fish flashed its white belly and soft brown body onto the scene. As it came into focus, I realized it wasn't another shark; it was a catfish! This bottom dweller of a fish wiggled its whiskers along the delicate organs in my body, slowly scanning every inch, and carefully sucked the leftover tiny crumbs into its soft mouth. Never blinking an eye, this fish moved as slow as an inchworm with the determination and discernment of a marine. I watched in amazement as I came to a conscious understanding of the significance of this shift in my meditation ritual. I blinked through tears and tasted the salt as they ran down my joyful face. In those intense moments, I experienced the power of the mind-spirit connection, which fed my body and soul with fuel for the next round of chemo.

Daily I prayed, and daily I meditated on Sharky and the catfish. Several days after the catfish came to mind, my husband drove me through the rush hour traffic to my fourth chemotherapy treatment. I glanced at Sharky on the dashboard and rubbed its little forehead with my index finger. Then out of nowhere, I had the urge to scratch my chest. As I reached up to scratch, my cell phone buzzed. It was a text message from my brother. "Pick it and flick it. Good luck on round four," it said. My chest itched again, and I felt sticky. I felt like my mind was going bonkers for a minute as I reread the message…Pick it and flick it…I pulled my iPod earbuds out of my ears, looked at my hubby, and said, "This is going to look weird, but I have to do this!" He said, "Whatever you have to do, honey, just do it!"

I closed my eyes, leaned back in the car seat, and let the spontaneous meditation flow. I reached up to scratch my scar and I "saw" and "felt" a gooey, sticky, honey-like mess spilling out of my chest. I clutched at the honey and started to pull it out of me, sticky long strings stuck between my fingers and my body. I felt like Sharky and the catfish had literally melted the tumor! As I pulled and stretched a handful, I tried to roll it and ball it up in my fingertips. I balanced a ball of the honey on my thumb, perched my index finger behind it, and flicked it as hard as I could out the car window. The honey poured out as I plucked and clutched with both hands, picking and flicking it all the way to the Cancer Institute.

A Sentence I Thought
I Would Never Say

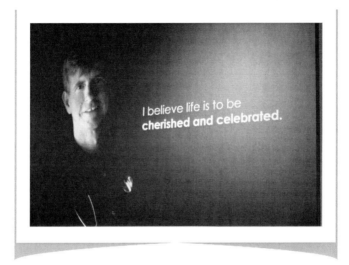

I believe life is to be
cherished and celebrated.

Photo by the author

Dr. Bob Reynolds, my oncologist, who
always knew just what to say to me.

RX: "A wise man's heart guides his mouth,
and his lips promote instruction. Pleasant
words are like honeycomb, sweet to the soul and
healing to the bones" (Proverbs 16:23–24).

I t was the last sweltering day of July, and I thought to myself, *It's about time!* The faster the days went by, the sooner my chemo would be over! Round five was done. This round I felt exhausted even before the adriamycin hit my veins. To top it off, I couldn't sleep that night. I was in bed by ten o'clock, I finished reading *Twilight*, and I finally turned the lights out at midnight; I woke up at 1:30. I moved to the family room couch. I was hungry by 2:00 a.m, so I ate a bowl of Banana Crunch cereal. Since my mind was awake and alive and nourishment was digesting in my intestines, I took notes regarding a work project and read half of a new 277 page book! Still awake at 4:00, I moved into our living room and curled up in our overstuffed, khaki green-colored chair and read for another thirty minutes. Craving the comfort of a bed, I crawled back in between the sheets and finally slept until around 6:00. I counted down the minutes until 7:00, which seemed like a much more reasonable time to finally give up on waiting for the sandman, and I rolled out of the bed.

It was a sticky, hot, sweaty-as-a-bees-knees day, not a cloud in the sky, with several more months of heat in the forecast. Since the heat and humidity were unusually uncomfortable for me that spring and summer, I decided to become a mall walker to get the walking exercise that I craved. Although it was ninety-five degrees outside, as I speed-walked past a Hallmark store, what before my wondering eyes did appear? Hallmark was unveiling its latest Christmas ornament collection for the upcoming holiday season! Normally in the summer, I ignored the fake snowflakes in the store windows and blazed past them, muttering to myself that time needed to slow down. I wanted to first feel the heat of the current season, then transition into the less humid, lovely fall days, enjoy the spirit of football season, Halloween, and Thanksgiving, and lastly, culminate into the joyous days of the reminder of Jesus's birth, silver bells, and red and green everywhere! Since Christmas seems to arrive earlier and earlier in the merchandise industry each year, I had trained myself to put on blinders and to not glance at the inflatable Santas and snowmen at Lowe's in August. In September, I didn't want to think about buying Christmas cards or wrapping paper or to look at Crate and Barrel's holiday catalog. In the past, by the time October and early November came around, I still ignored the aisles of strings of LED lights, "bigger and better" fake balsam wreaths, and shiny globes with angels in them. This year, however, even in July, I was mesmerized by the twinkling lights, the brightly colored decorations, and the thought that Christmas was on its way! By my calculation, I knew that this year, when Christmas was over and it wasn't quite the New Year, that this illness would all be over for me. Treatment for cancer would be a thing of the past. Lymphoma could become a memory. So in the heat of summer, sweat rolling down my forehead, I drove home from the mall, called my family, and announced one sentence I thought I would never say in July: "I can't wait for Christmas to come!"

My family and friends probably thought I was crazy, but as the summer and fall went on, I stopped and looked at Christmas decor wherever I was—Target, the pharmacy, Costco, the mall, you name it! The irony didn't escape me that celebrating the birth of Christ was coming at the same time I felt like I would be reborn. I hoped that I would come out of this incredible interruption of my life with new eyes. New hope was going to be born! I had survived the transition of moving from my mundane doctor and Holly-world to becoming a patient, and after Christmas, I would have to transition back. No one prepared me for that. Later, I would discover that it took courage and patience to find my way up a new learning curve and through the murky border between the worlds of no cancer and cancer and then back again to no cancer, but before that day came, I would just have to wait 'til Christmas!

None of us ever think anything awful or sad will happen to us or to our loved ones. Sure, we know the possibility is there, but we generally tend to feel immortal, invincible. We have all been on the listening end of a sad story, and virtually all of us know someone who either has/had cancer or was related to someone who has/had it. According to the American Cancer Society website, in January 2006, 11.4 million Americans with cancer or a history of cancer were alive. About 1.5 million new cancer cases were expected to be diagnosed in 2010. Cancer is the second most common cause of death in the United States (with heart disease being number one). That year alone, 569,490 Americans were expected to die of cancer: a rate of more than 1,500 of our loved ones per day! A little less than one in two men and a little more than one in three women will be diagnosed with cancer in their lifetime. These statistics are mind-blowing. Although the majority of us know someone who has been diagnosed with cancer, none of us ever really believe we will someday be told, "You are one of those 11.4 million." That is a hard sentence to hear or to say, so I'd rather be saying something else I thought I would never say, such as,

"I just won $500 million in the lottery!"

"I am playing on the US Olympic volleyball team!"

"I am moving to Hawaii to surf for a living!"

"An agent spotted me in the grocery store and wants me to do a photo shoot for the next issue of *Glamour* magazine!"

These are all prime examples of sentences I probably would never *say* and be telling the truth. I never imagined I would become a cancer patient, but I did. I had a stellar oncologist and team to help guide me through treatments and ultimately to recovery. My physician had a lot of wonderful words to say to me.

Here are some sentences I thought I would never *hear* in my lifetime. When I was in the hospital after my surgeries, my oncologist started to say, "You have Hodgkin's and that means—"

I was too scared to hear what he was going to say next, so I interrupted him and said emphatically, "I don't want to hear about my chances or percentages or—"

He then interrupted me reassuringly with these words, "Holly, we're going to cure you."

Then, one time at a follow-up appointment, I complained that I was tired, yet he said the best words—one of my favorite sentences—my ears could ever hear: "You are the healthiest person I will see today!"

Lastly, my nurse practitioner also seemed to always know what I needed to hear as well. Although I never imagined I would be on the receiving end of the words she used, she told me with sincerity in her eyes, "Your cancer team will make this nonsensical tumor go away. You are fine, better than fine!"

The power of language and the importance of saying the right thing at the right time never seemed as crucial to me as they did during this year. I also learned that the best conversationalists understood that sometimes silence was golden. Sometimes it was better to just say nothing at all to me. Just sit and be with me. That was enough! One word, one sentence could fill me up, or make me come crashing down. I loved hearing things like, "You look amazing!" and "You are an inspiration!" These quips made feel beautiful and strong and fearless!

On the other hand, I hated hearing questions like, "How is your hair doing?" Whenever someone asked me about my hair, I felt vulnerable. I was upset that someone was more concerned about my hair than my feelings about my hair. I wanted to reply with a smile if I could, "Thanks for asking. My oncologist styles it every other week!" I also couldn't stand to hear statements like, "You don't look like you have cancer." The response I wanted to give to that one? "Yet I know that I do have cancer, you want to know why? Because I have to go now..." (And here is the sentence I really thought I would never, ever say and be telling the truth.) "I have an appointment with my oncologist!"

Burnin' Sternum

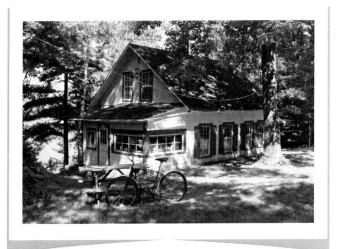

Photo by the author

The beloved Belle Acres.

RX: Envision pain as a sign of
weakness leaving the body.

t was dinnertime in the heat of the summer in the mid-1980s at Belle (pronounced "Belly") Acres in Rhinelander, Wisconsin. I was growing up and growing into my skin. Fried bluegill and bass crackled in the oil of the cast-iron grill pan, the bratwurst hissed over the coals, and my grandmother set out a dish of her famous wood-burning oven baked potatoes sprinkled with Mrs. Dash.

She called out to me to ring the dinner bell. The heavy, silver-colored dinner bell was attached to the trunk of a massive, old, magnificent oak tree about six feet up; a yellow nylon rope was attached to the clapper. I grabbed the rope and start ringing in my cousins and brother who were down the hill on the pier or somewhere close by in the woods. My aunt's spastic wire-haired terrier with its little muscular body and white hair flecked with orange and gray and brown wanted in on the action. Legs pumping, she somehow bounded up the tree trunk, situated her legs parallel to the ground and body vertical to the tree, grabbed the nylon rope in her jaws, and started flailing away. Her head was moving in a spasm of side-to-side movements—rapid fires of *Clang! Clang! Clang! Clang!* rang in our ears! I was in stitches, laughing hysterically, acutely aware of this never-seen-before talent of this mangy mutt! The dog's head then slowed to a trancelike state, and her body started quivering as she tired herself out and finally came down from the tree. The boys came running as the bell stopped ringing, and finally, it was time to eat after a long day of hiking on "Toad Road," running the length of the pier, hitting the water feet first, and rowing the old boat to "Turtle Bay" and "The Secret Fort."

There were only a few rules of etiquette at mealtime at Belle Acres: If you don't fish, you don't eat. Eat fast, so you get more. If food falls on the ground, you've got five seconds to eat it or likely your cousins will beat you to it! Any inedible leftovers like eggshells, gristle, potato skins, or apple cores go straight into the worm bed, not the trash. Oh, and don't confuse the hummingbird juice with the Kool-Aid, which to the delight of my giggling brother, I accidentally did once!

Summertime was sweet on Long Lake at Belle Acres with my dad's side of the family. The dirt and gravel road to the house was a quarter of a mile long, weaving between dense trees of our family's tree farm. The road opened up to a white summer cottage with red trim and a red roof, nestled into a steep hill; hand-dug, earthen steps led down to the shore of the lake. The front porch of the house had an old-fashioned wooden screen door, which made a delightful banging noise even when you tried to shut it quietly. Standing on the porch was an old, wide, white Frigidaire where my grandma kept the hummingbird juice. Next to the refrigerator was a huge tin cooler sitting high on a narrow table. There was a red button to push on the cooler and out poured fresh spring water, and I do not mean Zephyrhills or Poland Ice! (We were living so far into the boonies that we collected fresh water from a roadside fresh spring on our way into town!) Above and to the right of the cooler, a dented tin cup with a rolled lip hung from a long nail. It was the community cup from which we all drank summer after summer, year after year! Turning around on the front porch, looking toward the outside and the worm bed, the windowsills were lined with red and white bobbers, fishing nets, and dust—lots of dust.

These sweet childhood memories of the summers spent on Long Lake in Rhinelander, Wisconsin, are part of the fabric that shaped me. There are now new fibers sewn into that creation, and those fibers were spun during the scorching summer of cancer treatment in Winter Springs, Florida. That summer took on a different meaning, but it was still one of growing into my skin. It was a lifesaving summer with its own memories. As my brother called it—rather than the dog days of summer—it was the summer of the burnin' sternum.

In just a day after my first chemo Thursday and Neulasta Friday, I was walking around the block with my husband (smelling like a wet dog but only to myself, thank goodness!) *Where did that come from?* I wondered. Anyway, I felt my ribs and sternum become sore, achy, and tight; a very different sensation than my postoperative muscle soreness, and I realized that the Neulasta must be doing its job: building new marrow! I told my chemo nurse, "Katina, I feel like the sun is coming out of my chest!" Within four to six hours after each time I received that injection pinch in the back of my right upper arm, my chest felt like it was being knit together with hot needles; I could feel what felt like fibers weaving themselves together inside of me like a giant quilt being pulled tight on a loom. The skin overlying my chest and the bone of my sternum felt taut and warm, sort of like when you lay down at night after a day of sunburn. It was such a constrictive feeling that, for months, I couldn't stand the feeling of having on a bra or a tight shirt as that would just squeeze me more! I tried to wear a bra to my treatments to appear as normal as possible, but before I could get home, I would pull myself out of the confining boob-slinging apparatus and breathe a bit easier!

Often the ache in my bones would be concentrated at the base of my skull and top of my spine as well. I willed the burning feeling to be a sign of healing. "Pain is a sign of weakness leaving the body," someone once said to me. I believed her. Each treatment that came and went, the Neulasta kicked my bone marrow into hyperdrive, and my white blood cell count was sent soaring, often close to 40,000 (normal is from 4,300 to 10,800)! Sometimes the pain became so intense as my body repaired itself and protected itself against infection that I felt like I was being beaten by an Olympic personal trainer—however, with no physical rewards such as some coveted toned biceps or sleek, strong thighs, darn it!

While my sternum was on fire, my taste buds were also tricked out from the side effects of the medications. I often had to nibble on things I normally wouldn't let enter my mouth in order to just taste something besides a mixture of bad breath and metal! I relied on Lemonheads and watermelon Jolly Ranchers so my saliva didn't have to taste like a mouth that spent twenty-four hours without toothpaste. One afternoon after a chemo treatment, I was drinking glass after glass of water to hydrate. As the day wore on, the continually refilled cup of plain, calorie-free, filtered water started to taste weird. I didn't like it. I forced myself to keep drinking, making a face with every swallow. Finally after six or seven hours of the cycle of sip, horrible flavor, scrunch face, swallow, I looked at the bottom of the glass and saw a white, granular material. *What was in my water!?!* It took me a few minutes to figure out that I must have dropped a tablet of Tylenol into the glass earlier in the day! It had dissolved in the water, and the entire afternoon, I had been tasting, not the effects of chemo, but rather my own fumble of acetaminophen! I was laughing in relief when finally, the next glass of straight-up water on the rocks tasted just like, well, water!

During the summer of the burnin' sternum when my chest felt like the summer solstice and when my taste buds were not my own, I longed for water from the tin cup, fried fish, and bratwurst in Belle Acres. And so I dreamt of lying in the canoe in the middle of Long Lake, water gently sloshing the sides, waiting to hear the family pet ringing that darn dinner bell.

Eden: The Haircut

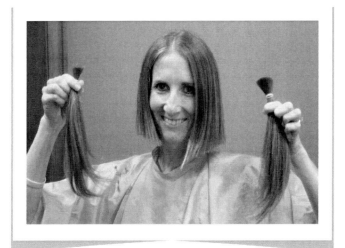

Photo by Nancy Woodruff

Four long ponytails were donated to Pantene's Beautiful
Lengths to make wigs for bald cancer patients.

RX: Keep your head where your feet are. Realize
that everyone is struggling with something.

I am a redhead. When I was growing up, I hated my hair. I was the only one in school from kindergarten through high school who had red hair. "Carrot top" and "Holly, Holly, Hobbie Doll" were sung around me as I walked the halls. When I went to slumber parties with a group of screaming, excited middle school girls to watch the Miss America pageant, my friends told me that I could never be Miss America because I had red hair; and Miss America never was a redhead they informed me. When I arrived back at home, crying, my mom told me that they said this mean thing because they were all jealous of my beautiful hair. I never quite believed her. However, eventually, I embraced my locks of rosy sunshine as it made me stand out from the sea of blonds and brunettes. If someone asked a friend of mine, "Did you see the girl with red hair?" The answer was always an easy, "Oh, yes. That was my friend, Holly!" I guess you could say that my long red hair became my best feature and that I was known for it. It was a part of my identity.

When I was told that 100 percent of patients on the chemotherapy medicine called Adriamycin, (the Jesus juice) would have their follicles stunned and lose their hair, I decided to be proactive and chop my locks before they started to fall out. The morning I decided to call the Eden Spa, the hair salon affiliated with the Cancer Institute at Florida Hospital, was difficult. It was four days after my first chemotherapy dose. I had pain from my surgery, and my stomach was in knots. I woke up and prayed in bed while the first dose of Percocet passed over my lips. I waited for the pain to pass and my morning poop to come. I knew within an hour of these three new morning rituals (the three Ps—pray, Percocet, and poop) I would feel better, and that brought peace. Once I did feel more like myself, I went for a walk around the neighborhood, and I thought about walking around bald. Then I took another lap, and I thought about walking around with a scarf on my head. Then I lapped for the third time, and I thought about walking around with a wig. *I could get a blond wig and finally be Miss America!* I finally got up the nerve to call the salon for a haircut and wig consultation for the next day. It was a moment of pure anxiety for me. I kept telling myself these four things:

1. I am getting a haircut tomorrow. I am not losing my hair tomorrow.
2. This is only temporary, just like my temporary tattoos.
3. My true beauty lies deep within, not in the long strands of strawberry hair on my head.
4. My best girlfriend Nancy will take me and be at my side during this external transformation I was about to face. I would not be alone.

After making the phone call, I read an article in a magazine about a man who was diagnosed with pancreatic cancer. His oncology nurse stated, "Keep your head where your feet are." In other words, stay in the moment; live one hour at a time. Appreciate the little things, the things you normally take for granted. The patient with cancer then said, "Everyone keeps telling me that cancer makes you appreciate the little things. But I have always appreciated the little things. What cancer really does is make you more aware that almost everyone is struggling with something." How very true, sir, very true. My redhead thinking cap now back into focus, I realized that I needed to add fun into this part of my journey. This was a moment for me to embrace my inner beauty and show people that all redheads don't have a temper but rather that this one had a sense of humor and a strong sense of self. I also made the decision to cut enough length of hair to donate to an organization that would use my hair to make wigs for other women or children who lost their hair due to cancer treatment. I realized my loss (of hair) would make someone else very happy, and that made me happy too!

I was fired up after reflecting on the good that could come out of a simple haircut, and so I sat and I wrote my top ten reasons for chopping the locks:

10. It was time to try something new and fun. (Ironically, I was not brave enough without cancer to go through with this kind of haircut.)
9. This was my chance to buy a pink wig just like Frenchie in the movie *Grease*.
8. I could reveal my inner goddess and inner biker chic!
7. I would have fewer gray hairs.
6. In the spirit of "Go Green," I would be using less shampoo and water.
5. This new cut would keep my neck cool just in time for the heat of the Florida summer.

4. Who doesn't love a bald icon with a lollipop hanging out of her mouth?
3. This would be the ultimate time and money saver. No shaving time, no bikini waxes at the salon, no hairstyling aids needed from the drug store, and no hair drying, curling, or straightening time in the morning!
2. I would be just like my new peer group, my chemo posse, and I would therefore fit in.
1. The opposite of aging would happen right before my eyes. It would be like reverse puberty!

With my top ten list in my pocket, I was ready to chop off the locks. I was planning to cut off eight inches, enough for me to donate, enough for me to have a cute chin-length cut, and a chance for a second cancer haircut when I was really shedding. I thought it would be less drastic for me if I made the cut in two different phases. The morning of the first cut Nancy was on time and smiling ear to ear as she and Shane took pictures of my long hair from all angles. Shane ran his fingers through my hair and held my face and told me what a brave thing I was doing. Then it was time to go.

The Eden Spa was serene yet hip and light and bright. I was led to a room that had a wall full of do-rags and wigs and a wig consultant. For over an hour, we talked about the pros and cons of real versus synthetic hair pieces, European locks, fun on-the-go looks, wigs that were sewn into baseball caps, wigs attached to headbands, and fuzzy night caps to keep my head warm once I became hairless. I tried on wigs of all colors and lengths and styles while Nancy clicked away with the camera. I threw my head back and posed and smiled and felt like a diva getting ready for a performance.

As I slipped the last wig off my head, a reality moment hit me about why I was there and what was about to happen. I started to bawl. The wig consultant folded me into her arms and stroked my hair, and Nancy hugged me tight. *Everyone is struggling with something. Keep your head where your feet are.* I was ready to roll.

My beautiful, long, red hair, my old identity, was divided into four ponytails and the hairstylist's sharp, silver scissors came out. One at a time—*snip, snip, snip, snip*—my ponytails were cut. I held them in my lap, and I looked up into the mirror. I expected to lose it again. Instead, I felt amazing! I felt liberated, I felt brave, I felt alive, I felt freedom! I looked adorable with my new chin-length cut! I had conquered one of my worst fears on this journey! Of course, the more fearful day would be the day that the hairs fell out of my head and were not just being cut off my head; but in that moment inside of Eden, I was feeling a little bit of heaven on this side of earth.

After the third chemotherapy treatment, I had a follow-up appointment with my oncologist. Everything was going as planned, my blood tests looked good, I was feeling just like they told me I would feel going through the chemo treatments, and I was told that I needed to plan on six full months of chemo (not four as he had mentioned as a possibility early on in my treatment plan). I told my doctor, "I only want to fight this monster once, and if that means six months of chemo will decrease the chance of it going away and never coming back, then six months it is!" Since everything seemed to be going as expected, he asked me if I had encountered any surprises along the way. I only paused for a second before answering, "Yes, there is!"

He looked at me curiously, tilted his mop of red hair, and asked, "What is that?"

With glee and a smile on my face, I said, "I still have my hair!"

He assured me that it was just a matter of time before I didn't have my hair, but I'll tell you what, reader, every day that I woke up and my hair was still tight on my scalp, I thanked God that on that day, I had hair! I no longer pulled out my stray gray hairs, and if I was having a bad hair day, I didn't care, because I still had hair!

As things go, two days later, my hair really started to shed a lot. Brushing and drying my hair that day was heart wrenching. I sat on the bathroom floor, and with my bare hands, I pulled the strands out of my brush and off the floor and into the garbage can. The tears came as I struggled with the reality of the inevitable. If you looked at me at that moment sitting Indian-style on the tile of the floor with the hair swept up, however, you would never know that I was losing my hair. I had to tell myself that when I finally did shave my head and go bald, it would only be for a short time and that it would be for the greater good. I wanted my cancer to go away, and if that meant my hair had to go away, too, let it fall!

I must have had a lot of hairs per square inch on my head. I made it through eight out of twelve treatments before I couldn't take the waterfall of strands that cascaded out of my follicles into the hairball-river at my feet any longer. I didn't like the feeling of the strands getting knotted up in between my toes as I walked across the carpet. I didn't like the feeling of palmfuls of wet hair coming out in the shower as I rinsed away the Finesse shampoo. I didn't like seeing my scalp through the thin strands of red chemo-hair that was left on my head. The day had finally come. I was ready for a new challenge. Here comes baldy!

On a Saturday afternoon, sacrificing the 3:30 college football game kickoffs, my husband drove me to a salon. I wore all my power bracelets and sat on the couch in the art-deco waiting room. While we waited, the hairstylist's little white terrier dog invited himself up onto my lap and promptly fell asleep. The stylist was amazed as her dog had never done that before with any of her clients. It seemed that this dog, like Biscuit, knew I needed some extra love. When it was my turn, I sat up high in the salon swivel chair. A dark brown ivy-patterned smock was tightened around my neck, and my hair was again divided into a bunch of small ponytails. I was hoping to donate even more! One at a time each ponytail was lopped off and put into my lap. Then my hair was cut into a pixie-do only about an inch long, and I had cute little sideburns! The stylist corrected me when I mentioned the sideburns. She said, "Those aren't sideburns. Those are your personalities!"

My alter ego was no longer screaming to get out; I was a real biker chic now—short hair, tattoos, personalities, and I had a new surprise for everyone around me. I never lost all of my hair. Ahhh, Eden.

Army of Angels

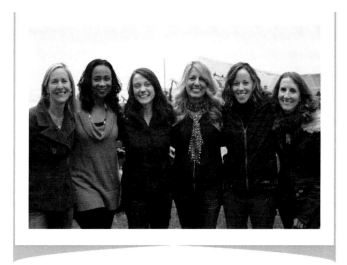

Photo by Ray Fiechter

Celebrating with my Ya-Yas (Shari, Nikki, Shantel, Nancy, Kathy, and me) in Indianapolis.

RX: Gather your friends.

Within days of the whirlwind of my diagnosis, I was not only overwhelmed with the thoughts of surviving cancer, I was also overwhelmed with the incredible support of family, friends, and acquaintances. Even though my husband and my mom held my hands through the initial tornado and my brother kept me laughing, I also needed my friends. When I needed prayer, I called Shari. When I needed encouragement, I called Shantel. When I needed someone to sit with me in the moment, I called Nancy. And when I needed to express myself through writing, I sent mass sentiments and photos through e-mail to friends all over globe.

Preacher and author, Leroy Brownlow writes,

> The need for friends is imperative. It is not good for us to be friendless. We were made to give and to receive, to help and to be helped, to encourage and to be encouraged, to feel and bond with others. Standing alone can never satisfy. Our nature requires a tie to faithful others. We call it friendship.

I love my friends, and I knew this experience might strengthen some ties, break some others, and make some new ones. As sure as God was the lifeblood in my marrow, my friends and family were the skeleton doing everything they could do to support me and help me to stay upright!

Whether fighting for your life, your job, your marriage, or your country, you will find that there is strength in numbers. When I found the elephant in my chest, the first person I told when I got home from work was my husband; although the support of my significant other was crucial for me, the second person I recruited was my mom. I then drafted my brother, father, stepfather, my close circle of friends, my pastor, other family members, my boss, and my workmates. As word spread, friends and family volunteered to be on "Team Holly." Overwhelmed by the love of others, I began to communicate my battle stories and victory songs in mass e-mails to what I called my Army of Angels. Thriving on words of encouragement from so many people, I learned quickly it would be impossible to "go it alone." I admit, e-mailing stories with my health updates, my thoughts, my feelings, and photos were selfish in many ways. Although friends and family wanted to know what was happening through my eyes, I also wanted e-mails of encouragement back! On top of God's peace and my ability to find hope in His arms, I also needed to know that people cared about me enough to send a kind word. I thrived on receiving this support! Through these e-mails, I received great advice and encouragement, and I shared some of my deepest thoughts and feelings. In doing this, I generated instant emotional and spiritual therapy for myself, completely free of charge! I was also grateful for family and friends loving me a thousandfold when I wasn't able to give much back.

Before I even had the final diagnosis, one of my angel encouragers, Shantel, said to me, "This could be the best and biggest interruption in your life. There is no change without conflict. Along with these interruptions come discoveries." Although I didn't want change or conflict, these words gave me a peace beyond my own comprehension that something good was about to come out of the looming elephant in my chest! I discovered that God does indeed disturb us when we are comfortable, and then He turns around and comforts us when we are disturbed. There was a gradual unraveling of truth in her wisdom. I now pass on these wise words to others who are about to embark on the ride of their lives.

When I was nervous about my chest being sawed opened and put back together, and how the scarring and healing would change the looks of my body, another encouraging friend, who happens to be a breast cancer survivor, empathized with me. She said that whenever she sees her scars, they are her reminder that yes, "life is hard, but God is good." When I heard that, I thought to myself, *Wow! She just spread the love of God in seven short words. Think of how I will be able to encourage others with my very own scars!*

After my third treatment, I was having a difficult morning as my hair was falling out as fast as rain from a cloud and landing on the bathroom floor. Shane came and sat with me on the tile where I was bawling. I asked him if he would still love me when my hair all fell out, and he said, "Honestly? I will love you more." I then had to go to work later that day, and while I was in the car on the way, Shane called my nurse to tell her that I had had a hard morning and that I might need a hug when I got there. Not only did I get several hugs, my workmates also bought me a vanilla Steak-N-Shake milkshake and pampered me for the next four hours.

"Sit down, Dr. Johnson," "Go get a snack," and "I'll get it, Dr. J" were sentences I heard throughout my shift. I was certainly on the receiving end of "in sickness and in health" from Shane that day!

Besides encouragement, I also received much needed advice from the Army of Angels. The following survival story comes from my aunt, a thyroid cancer survivor, who wrote:

> I was admitted to the hospital in isolation, and radiation was injected into me. It was very dramatic...I had to be encased in lead aprons, and no one was allowed in or out of the room except the doctors and head shift nurses...For three days I remained in isolation with a drip and forcing fluids like crazy...A doctor came in daily to wave a Geiger counter over me to see the progression of the radiation. My pee was captured in a special toilet, and I was served food on paper products...there was even a ring painted on the floor around the bed, and only the doctors and nurses stepped in the ring!

I figured anyone who could endure three days of isolation in lead aprons, confined to a painted ring on the floor was worth getting advice from! Therefore, the following is a list of advice from my aunt, Dr. Denise:

1. Do what the doctors tell you to do...don't second guess them.
2. Take all of your medications on time.
3. Keep all of your appointments, and be early. (Editor's note: You never know who you might

meet in the waiting room that will become a friend for life.)

4. Don't fight sleep!
5. Try hard to not be crabby with anyone.
6. Work, work, and then work some more. (Editor's note: This advice is not for everyone!)
7. Finally, do not listen to what other people have experienced! Everyone reacts differently, and there is not a set course for anything such as this. (Editor's note: My aunt and I heard horrible stories from other survivors and well-meaning family and friends, none of which we experienced.)

During my convalescent time, I not only received oodles of advice and words of encouragement from others, I also had plenty of my own thoughts during this extra free time I was handed. In an e-mail to a missionary friend in Ghana, I wrote:

> You know something that I have realized…I knew it before, but now I really see it…and have been amazed by, is the presence of God in all of our lives at all times in all places at any moment. He has us—you and me—fully in His hands without cheating either of us. He is that awesome and incredible that He can make each of us feel like we are the only ones standing before Him and praising Him, questioning Him, and talking to Him. And He does that all at once; talk about the ultimate multitasker!

The Angels often asked me how I was coping, and I would pass on a story I once heard about a man lost at sea floating around for days who was ultimately rescued. People later asked him what he thought about all day floating around, God knows what lurking under the waves, and salt water beneath him. Wasn't he scared, anxious, doubtful that he would ever be rescued? He simply said that what got him through was that he concentrated on seeing God only. That was what I was doing as I woke up every day and went on with living...I just concentrated and saw God only. He sent me an inspiring Army of Angels to draw strength from; I call them my cosurvivors. I truly feel we became one voice standing against my cancer—the line between me and the angels was blurred. In an e-mail to the Army before my last chemo dose, I wrote, "Can you believe it? *We* are almost done!"

Every "bone" in my body, every member of the Army of Angels, has remained strong while going up the river and down the river and through the wildest storm to date in my life. I am blessed and lucky. Family and true friends are golden in the time of being pressure-cooked. My cancer mantra may have been from Job 23:10, "Although He has tested me, I shall come forth as gold," but one thing that I know for sure is that I have come forth *with* gold, and gold equals friends.

Bartley's and Blueberries

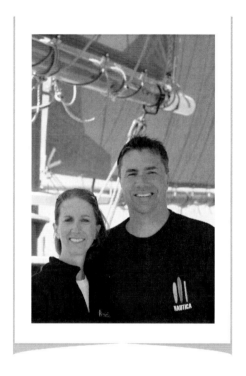

Photo by random tourist on board our ship

On *The Margaret Todd* schooner in Bar Harbor, Maine.

RX: Rediscover yourself. Take a trip.

With Project: Tumor Annihilation and Mission: Remission under my belt after round 4, I retreated to the corner of the boxing ring for a water break and bandaging. *Who was I? Where did I go? How can I find myself again?* My once carefree life was now defined by doctor's appointments every week, blood draws, a healing chest wound, and crazy red pee. I wasn't sure I had any say-so about decisions in my life or any personal preferences about anything anymore! I felt lost! I had to go in search of my soul and mind. Luckily, I found them again while biting into a really juicy hamburger in Cambridge and in a slice of sinfully sweet blueberry pie in Acadia. This is the story about a trip to the Northeast and how I found myself again...

After a long travel day, my husband and I were in our gray Chevy Cobalt rental car, with Sharky on the dashboard, on the way through the winding roads of Boston in search of our bed and breakfast. Finding the inn was a great adventure, like searching for a needle in a haystack called the "Big Dig," the nickname the locals gave to the road construction. The roads in the city go every which way but straight to your destination, and none of the streets were well-marked, but eventually, our car pulled up to the charming B&B. Our room was decorated with white walls, two double beds with shiny lime-green bedspreads, black-and-white photos on the walls, and a very small bathroom. Our view of Massachusetts Avenue was obstructed by a big beautiful tree with limbs that chased after each other and tickled the windowpanes.

Once we checked in, we drove a few miles into Harvard Square and set out on foot to the campus of Harvard. It is a beautiful campus, and I could feel the history and tradition oozing out of the buildings. The campus is surrounded by high, black wrought-iron fences and gates. The main square on campus is surrounded by larger-than-life brick dormitories. Deeper into the campus is a beautiful white brick church. Directly opposite is an enormous library with high and wide concrete steps—a formidable-appearing learning institute. Their stacks must go on for miles! I felt smarter just by sitting on the steps.

We stumbled upon the Harvard Bookstore, which was full of the character of an old-time book market with wooden shelves zigzagging throughout the floor plan, nooks and crannies full of periodicals, words, book spines, and knowledge. Downstairs was chock-full of bargains, and poles supporting the ceiling were plastered with comics and witty comments placed by many people over the years. I bought a $6.50 Maya Angelou bargain book and was beaming walking out of there!

A skip and a jump down the sidewalk, I discovered Mr. Bartley's, a local favorite hamburger joint that got my heart pumping the minute I stepped inside. Every family style table and seat was filled with young people and loud voices. The walls were full of crazy stuff like bumper stickers, Elvis posters, an old Ronald Reagan ad for cigarettes, and a Star Trek postcard. Over the cooking area hung a huge blackboard with the burger menu. Their burgers had names like The Bill Clinton, The Tom Brady, The John McCain, and The George Bush! Each burger topping was chosen to reflect the personality of its namesake. The place was altogether fantastic! After stuffing our faces with the thick, juicy burgers and piles of fries, we walked around outside.

I popped into Sweets! for a vanilla cupcake; we stood on the sidewalk with a handful of baseball fans and watched, on a TV inside of a store window, the Red Sox play the Yankees; we held hands and kissed under an enormous tree with strands of deep blue and purple lights…It was like a dream. I felt like coffee, percolating into myself again, and realizing I still did have likes and dislikes, I still could make my own choices, and I was alive and living life just fine, cancer or not!

After a restful night of sleep, we went to Fenway Park. The area surrounding the park was teeming with workers and fans. We grabbed a sandwich under the bleachers at a bar and grill, which looked out over centerfield toward the Green Monster and home plate. After lunch, we piled into the car and started the long drive along the coast, passing the New Hampshire and Maine state lines toward Bar Harbor.

The next morning we awoke to bright blue skies, cool weather, and blueberry yogurt and granola for breakfast. We popped into the rental car and drove to the main entrance to Acadia National Park. I am a huge fan of the National Park system, and seeing the traditional brown National Park sign made me giddy, kind of like coming home. We watched a short film about the history of the park at the Visitors Center. I learned that the forested and granite land and mountains of Acadia were entirely donated by wealthy families back in the days of the Vanderbilts and the Rockefellers who had the foresight to preserve that land for the generations who came long after they were gone. Miles of carriage roads with impressive granite-block bridges were constructed and hiking trails were forged. Autos were later allowed on the Park Loop Road, a twenty-seven-mile road, which we drove. Sharky led the way, and we stopped at multiple unique sites to Acadia including Sand Beach, Thunder Hole, and Cadillac Mountain.

Sand Beach is nestled between rocky cliffs and loud, pounding waves cresting and thundering at the shoreline. The beach was packed with families soaking up the rays and riding the surf of summer. Near the beach we saw a big black Newfoundland dog that had big, clumsy feet and was shaved except for a mohawk. That got a laugh from several people!

Thunder Hole is a gorgeous area of rocky cliffs and boulders, which congregate in such a way that as the tide comes in, especially on a stormy day, the surf enters a "hole," creating a vacuum effect until the tide rushes out then releases its energy with a loud *boom!* Since it wasn't storming and it wasn't high tide, however, we only heard some gurgling noises. Of greater interest was the scenery and the thrill of finding a special spot on the rocks to sit and to listen to the sea and look out over the coast.

On the recommendation of many strangers along the way, we stopped at Jordan Pond, had lunch, and indulged in their famous flaky, buttery popovers with real whipped butter and homemade strawberry jam. My taste buds were alive and happy as the baked goodie melted in my mouth. On the short hike to the pond, we passed through a blueberry field and had a taste of the tart Maine berry. We hiked along the pond on a gravel trail and drank in the scenery of the surrounding pine-filled hills.

The big finale of the day was the drive 1,500 feet up to the summit of Cadillac Mountain. We were blessed with a very clear day to see an almost 360-degree view of the surrounding area including Bar Harbor, the coast, and the other mountain ranges, which were formed by volcanic forces and moving glaciers millions of years ago. Off of the coast, we could see tens of green island clumps that look so traditionally "Maine." We shared a blueberry soda, letting the sweet, syrupy, carbonated beverage tingle on our tongues and hiked all over the top of Cadillac so we could drink in every view.

Back on Main Street in Bar Harbor, we passed by quaint shops each with their special shingle hanging overhead with funny names like "The Thirsty Whale," "Windowpane," and "The Moose Hole." We walked through a gathering square of fresh grass and a white gazebo on a hill that sloped gently toward the water overlooking the boats and the small islands offshore.

We were seated overlooking the pier and the waterfront at the Harbor Inn terrace with great anticipation of a lobsterfest! First we were brought a piping hot blueberry cornbread muffin and a thick, creamy bowl of clam chowder with oyster crackers. Then out came two bowls of dirty white clams with gray-yellow meat and dark mussels with orange-brown meat. These were served with a dipping bowl of broth and a second dipping bowl of melted butter. I attempted to pick at the meat of a clam, dipped it in the cloudy broth to remove the grit, dipped it in the golden butter, and put the ball of rubbery, mucousy meat in my mouth, determined to say that I tried a clam (!) but I couldn't do it! I couldn't stomach even just swallowing one!

Our waiter brought a bowl with our lobster bibs, wet wipes, napkins, shell crackers, and crustacean meat pickers. In the spirit of the lobsterbake, Shane donned the plastic bib that said, "Let's get crackin'!" Then, our bright-red one-pound lobsters were served in their full glory, beady eyes popping, along with corn on the cob and red potatoes. It was fun watching Shane dig in and learning how to tear off the lobster claws and get to the meat. The work of finally releasing the white-and-pink meat was actually more fun than eating it! (Note to self: I do not need to order lobster, clams, or mussels again!) The last course of the meal was delicious blueberry pie. The berries were tart and their taste was complemented by the thick, sweet, golden piecrust. We ended our evening by watching the apricot-orange moon rise and ambling back to our hotel.

After sleeping well on a very comfortable bed, we woke up to another perfect weather day, ate breakfast (blueberry pancakes, of course), and walked to the harbor for a cruise aboard a four-masted schooner called *The Margaret Todd*. The captain had two Newfoundland dogs, Maggie and Brig, who claimed their spots at the stern with the captain and the wheel. Shane got to help the crew raise the reddish, weather-beaten canvas sails with the call of "One, two, one, two!" We sailed in circles around the many islands in the harbor and saw plenty of lobster buoys and traps. The air on the water was cool and being on a boat with the swells of the sea around me, my soul was filled and my spirit cleansed. By late afternoon, the sun had set on our Bar Harbor/ Acadia adventure, and it was time to take the long drive back to Boston.

In Boston for the last day of our trip, we visited the John F. Kennedy Museum and Library. Since I am not a history buff, I was unsure about how much I would enjoy our time there, but I found myself fascinated, interested, and contemplative. The exhibits were displayed clearly and in a very organized fashion that told a story, purposely not focusing on the assassination, but rather on JFK's magnetic personality, his vigor for life and serving our country, and his beloved family.

Scurrying to see more of the city of Boston in a very limited time, we set out on foot on the bricked footpath of the Freedom Trail to Paul Revere's house, the Mall, the North Church, and some of the winding cobblestone streets along Little Italy. We walked through the Boston Common, an area of green refuge among the concrete and brick historical buildings. Kids were splashing in the Frog Pond fountain, families were sitting in the shade, and men dressed in period costume led tourist groups through the park. We ambled into Cheers and saw the bar that inspired the era "where everybody knows your name."

It felt great to take a drink called vacation. The trip was a great escape from the new, unfamiliar life I was leading that crazy summer. Vacation freed me from thinking and contemplating how I was physically feeling practically every moment of the day. It was a time of choosing things I loved to do each day and then carrying that out, taking sidesteps along the way. It was a time of drinking in new areas to explore, being along the water, enjoying fresh air, and being outdoors under the big, blue sky (without the Florida humidity)! Boston and Bar Harbor were places of living passionately with a chance to make every single day count. The vacation reminded me that yes, I am still *me*, solidly, graciously, deeply to the core *me*. This was an important discovery that, of course, had been there all along—it's just that the wave had washed ashore, and I rose up out of the glorious debris.

Shedding My Old Self

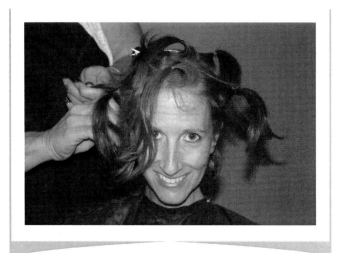

Photo by Shane Johnson

My second haircut during cancer
treatment. More red hair for wigs.

Rx: Be open for growth.

One afternoon after my one of my treatments I was looking out of our sliding glass doors into our backyard and across the pond; the green grass was stretching toward the sun, and on our cozy back patio a family of Florida lizards was making itself at home. They were scurrying around in the newly planted yellow marigolds, the society garlic, the ficus tree, and on our patio chairs and table. I noticed one rather large gray-brown lizard was doing its typical lizard push-ups on the black metal frame of the tabletop, its flaming orange-yellow neck gullet fanning in and out. In and out. In and out. Hypnotized by this moment, I saw that there was a fuzziness, a transparent white shroud about its neck, torso, and front legs. I blinked and I realized that it was molting! It was shedding the old, dry, dead skin and showing its tender but tough new exterior. Molting is a reptile's way of growing bigger than its old self. At many points in our lives, we all get that chance to grow bigger than our old selves, to develop into something new. For me that point was my cancer. I got a chance to shed my malignant cells and shine anew!

As chemotherapy melted the cancer from my body, another part of my treatment involved getting a shot of Neulasta growth factor that stimulated my bone marrow to produce more white blood cells. I was continually amazed at how my body responded to this medicine! Within four hours of that shot, I could literally feel the marrow in my sternum, in my ribs under my armpits, and in the vertebrae in the back of my neck start to make new cells! It was a deep stretching, burning pain like I was ready to burst out of my skin! Like the lizard, here I would go, making new "skin" to transform into a healthier, new body, different than the one twenty-four hours ago.

I have a new six-inch scar down the center of my lower sternum. My upper sternum is swollen and gives my chest a deformed look; I look like I have a pigeon's chest, sticking out like I do now. In my left upper chest, I have a one-inch scar and just below that underneath my skin on my skinny chest, there is a bump where my power port is. In my bilateral lower rib areas in front, I have two other healing scabs where the chest tubes were. My outer appearance—my exterior—is forever changed. Like my mind and spirit are being stretched to a new shape, so it is with my body as well.

We are constantly evolving, scanning, repairing, heart-beating, growling, digesting, sending impulses, inhaling, exhaling, fighting disease, building, blinking, tasting—the list is endless! We are so much more resilient than our mind can wrap around! With each molting session, we become a stronger, tougher, better version of ourselves, just for a time. And then it happens again and again, and we watch others go through it too, and we are all better for it. We are new.

Mission: Cure

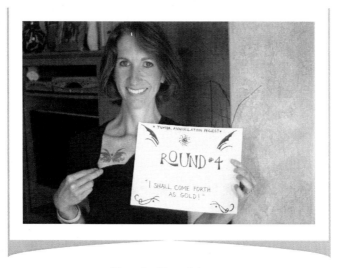

Photo by Shane Johnson

The Tumor Annihilation Project is ending.
Chemo treatment number four.

RX: Follow your intuition.

Seven days after chemo number four, I got to hear what every cancer patient longs to hear… But first I had to be scanned again from skull to thigh with a radioactive glow and thrown into what felt like a penalty box, eagerly looking to jump back into the ring, as I nervously waited for results.

The morning before I received a phone call from my tall, redheaded medical oncologist, I woke up early to go to the second PET scan appointment in my life. In the dark, my husband drove, and as the tires whirred on the pavement, I put in my earbuds and listened to the music that so far had carried me through the summer. Amazingly, I didn't feel anxious or nervous. When we arrived at the nuclear imaging site, I had to follow the same instructions as I did with my first PET scan. An IV was started in my arm, and I was asked to drink my first cup of contrast; it tasted like warm water with a touch of sweetness. Then the bubbly, spirited technician injected the IV contrast from the silver thermos into my arm. Next, the lights went out, and I rested under the stiff but warm hospital blankets quietly for an hour. Fifteen minutes before my scan, I drank the second cup of contrast. Then, off I went into the scan room! I felt dazed, and I had another moment when I felt like I was leading someone else's life, certainly not my own. At scan time, I covered my eyes with an eye mask that I had saved from a long airplane trip in my "previous life." I felt comforted. The scanner table was raised, and I slid into the machine's gut. With my eyes closed, I sang to myself, and I did what I had to do to soothe myself and not feel trapped and anxious. Occasionally

I would hear the hum of the machine, and unmoving, I waited patiently for the test to end. Twenty-five minutes later, I was back on my feet, being led to the waiting room where Shane was smiling and giving me a thumbs-up sign.

Elated to be done, but tired and hungry, we walked across the street to the Cancer Institute for an appointment with the nurse practitioner. My blood counts looked great, and the nurse reassured us that my tumor was "surely melting away." She kept saying, "I just love you guys. You don't need me! You are doing great!" After the appointment, it felt wonderful walking away from the hospital. It was good to be done with this step—the first PET scan after starting treatment. Now, all I had to do was wait for the official results.

Unofficially, I had a feeling that the tumor was massively shrinking. I felt this way because during my meditation sessions over the month prior, Sharky seemed to have vacated my chest! I just couldn't conjure him up. I felt like there was nothing left for him to chomp on; no matter how hard I concentrated on imagining his giant jaws gnawing away inside of me, he wouldn't appear. The catfish, however, remained and I would still envision him carefully scanning the environment in my chest and then eating the stray crumbs and scum. Then about three weeks before my scan when I sat down in the quiet to meditate on this God-given imagery, the catfish was putting on a disappearing act as well! I could picture it, bring it to mind, but the image would quickly dissipate. I thought to myself, *Could this mean that the tumor is gone?* I will never know if it was gone at that exact moment or not, but I was about to find out if it was there now.

The evening after my scan, I anxiously called one of the nurses at the Cancer Center who looked up the results of the scan on her computer. She started saying all these words that I wasn't really listening to, and then I heard the word "resolution." I interrupted her and said, "Wait! Don't you want Dr. Reynolds to see the report first and for him to tell me the rest?!?" She said that it was good news and she didn't want me to wait, so she continued to read the entire cancer-free news report. I was in shock, spellbound, and elated! I didn't have detectable cancer anymore! I felt like a miracle had just happened! After clutching Shane for several minutes, I was on my knees thanking God for this news—for my life!

Later, Dr. Reynolds called me, and the first words out of his mouth were "Holly, you are in remission!" Then, he said, "Go out and celebrate!" These were the words that I longed to hear two months ago when I first found the monster in my chest! In his ever calm, steady voice and caring nature, my doctor told me that patients with Hodgkin's who go into remission early are the ones who tend to be cured and that the cancer doesn't come back. He said that he would still stick to the twelve chemo treatment plan, plus radiation, and that he wanted to do another PET scan after the next four treatments. When I asked him, "Why?" He said, "Because I am a compulsive guy." He likes to follow protocols that work. He was saving my life, so how could I possibly argue with him? I felt like I wanted to run a marathon, and I had just been given a lifetime to do that! Mission: Remission accomplished…On to Mission: Cure!

Feeling It All

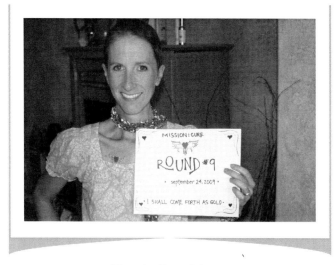

Photo by Shane Johnson

In remission during Mission: Cure. Treatment
number nine and coming forth as gold.

RX: Don't hold back.

In the beginning of my diagnosis and this incredible journey I told myself that I wanted to feel everything, really sit still and feel it, whether that meant pain or no pain, weakness or strength, joy of heart or heartache, a sweaty head or a cool breeze. Whatever I was feeling, I knew that God wanted it for me, in that particular moment, and with a purpose. It was hard when I was seeing my world through the lens of pain or anxiety, but I summoned my inner strength, grace, and sense of humor as best as I could on a given day and just went with it. I wanted to feel deeply and embrace my humanness and vulnerability and not to numb myself to my experience. Over one intense year, some things that I learned were what it was like to have really bad mornings, insomnia, pain, gratefulness, joy, hot flashes, and food cravings—no shortcuts! I intended to store these feelings so that my empathy and compassion for others would blossom. These experiences were laced with purpose, and I was not about to sit on the sidelines and feel sorry for myself! I wanted this to be a time of discovery and adventure—a story worthy to tell sitting around a kitchen table.

Twelve days after surgery and two days after my first chemotherapy treatment, I finally admitted that the mornings were difficult. I would wake up with pain, unable to get up at first, so I prayed in bed while a dose of Percocet passed my lips. I waited for the pain in my ribs, chest, and abdomen to pass and for my morning poop to come. It was then that I knew I would feel better after about an hour, and usually I did.

The simplicity of one Sunday was this: live one hour at a time, get out of bed, eat breakfast, shower, and get to church. It was communion Sunday, and I was grateful to participate. (Beware, reader, here comes some geeky doctor talk!) As I drank the grape juice and ate my cracker, I literally could feel the elements come alive in my mouth. I felt the soft tissues and tongue in my mouth prepare to swallow, followed by the gentle rhythm of peristalsis to move the food and drink down my esophagus to my stomach. They passed through my stomach valve and entered the world of my intestines. I imagined Christ nourishing me from within and taking out all that was bad in me.

I guess the powerful imagery, however, didn't last long on my good and healthy conscience. On the ride home, I had a sudden craving for a Filet-O-Fish sandwich, not the wisest, most nutritious selection I could have made. Actually, I didn't know what was going on with me during my early recovery time; I often got the strangest food cravings. I wanted bean burritos from Taco Bell, Lay's potato chips, mozzarella cheese sticks, deli-sliced turkey sandwiches, steak, milk chocolate, and dried apricots! I felt like what a hormone-laden pregnant woman must feel like! I am normally very particular about what I decide to swallow, so these outbursts of food insanity surprised me; but since my oncologist didn't want me to lose weight, and I had the cravings, I went along with them hoping that, like cancer, they were only temporary.

At times, I didn't know if I was feeling what pregnant women must feel with crazy food-cravings or feeling rather menopausal instead. About three months into my treatments, I stopped having my periods, and no, I wasn't pregnant! Soon after that, I started having hot flashes! They literally were like power surges of heat—a blast from an open oven door—that started from my scalp and worked its way to my ankles. I could tell when they were coming. It was as if an internal thermostat sounded an alarm. With the warning signal, I often had to strip down to a single layer of clothes or roll up my sleeves and pant legs. I started sweating within seconds of the alarm, the saltwater pouring from my sweat glands. In the first few days after chemo, whenever I had a hot flash, I swear I smelled like a wet dog. No one else ever confirmed that with me; maybe others just refused to come too close! The hot flashes lasted about two months. I had my last one on an airplane, coming home from Dallas. A mile high in the sky, I hoped in that moment that my periods would once again eventually return and regulate and that I would be back to being a normal thirty-nine to forty-year-old woman having monthly cycles! (I also thought, *God, I can't believe I just wished that on myself!*)

Cravings and hot flashes, I learned to live with. Pain, I did not. Yes, recovering from the pain of surgery was rough but expected. What I felt two months into chemotherapy, however, was certainly not. It was during this time that I had one of the worst pains I had ever had. The pain was sharp, intense, and then throbbing pain in my left shoulder blade area that radiated up to my shoulder and behind my left ear. It was so intense that I was in tears. I called off work for a couple of days and just lay in bed or on the couch. At the same time, I was also recovering from a head cold, and it felt like a sock was stuck in my upper nose…no fun when I was crying on top of the nasal congestion, trying to get a breath in between sobs! Like I stated, this pain was like nothing I had before. It was a different pain than the Neulasta pain, which I had learned to respect and appreciate. Every other treatment this new, unbearable pain seemed to come back. I would literally rock back and forth, my face wet with salty tears, counting down the minutes until I could take another pain pill.

Yet a different pain came after my first week in radiation. I got a surge of pain in my chest that felt like I would split open. It encircled my upper ribs and throbbed into my neck. I became exhausted in mind, body, and spirit; and it was showing. I started to crack easily rather than gracefully. Even when the pain improved, it became hard to swallow, especially cold water, and I often burped from the depths inside of me that made me feel like I was turning inside out. My protective tiny hairs in my airway became stunned from the radiation, and I had to cough more often as a result in order to sweep out the dust. Coughing, of course, only intensified the pain.

I was feeling it all—pain, anxiety, hopelessness, and fear (will it always be like this from now on?)—and I knew I had to help myself. I just refused to fall apart. I had to be the change I wished to see in my world (stated originally by Gandhi, edited by me to fit my circumstances)! I wanted to feel joy again. I prayed, I read from Psalms, and I used more visual imagery as

I listened to Hawaiian music while having radiation treatments. I visualized Ka'anapali Beach and the view overlooking the other islands from Maui. I told myself, I was in the soft sand, not the hard trilogy bed. I felt the aloha sun on my face, not the microwave rays of medicinal centigray. I squeezed my hand, holding an acorn I had placed there before my treatment, and I knew I was holding a gem.

> A symbol of strength,
> Change,
> Or potential, that helps us
> Realize the
> Newness of spirit and energy within.

Like an acorn, this pain had potential. I just had to learn to harness its energy before I finally could feel peace and serenity again and therefore grow and spread my roots and branches. This peacefulness then led to feelings of gratefulness whenever I had a pain-free day and gave me overflowing compassion for those living with chronic pain syndromes.

Another crazy thing that happened was that after chemo Thursdays and Neulasta Fridays, I couldn't sleep! After every treatment, I became an insomniac for two nights in a row! I attributed this wakefulness to the steroid therapy I was receiving that helped prevent nausea and helped boost the effects of my chemo. Sure, it was frustrating to not sleep at first because I was really tired after treatments, but I also noticed that I felt wired. (Tired but wired!) I was also strangely, happy... kind of tickled pink that this insomnia was happening.

Therefore I called it my joy'roid times! I would feel tired, lay in bed, and by 2:00 or 3:00 in the morning, still be wired! I would move to the couch, read hundreds of pages in the *Twilight* series of books, come up with new work ideas, or just eat. You see, the food cravings didn't just stop when the sun went down! Midnight snacks (and later) were common for me...nothing like a bowl of Banana Crunch cereal at 4:00 a.m.! Yum! I wish I could have that kind of happy energy all the time! I couldn't wait until the clock struck seven in the morning because that meant someone would be at my work by that time. I would call my workmates just so I could finally have someone to talk to after a restless night and no one to pass the time with. No one else was up at that hour, so again, I just went with it and made that phone call to the Army of Angels at work every other week!

Treatments weren't all bad; in truth, going to chemo were mostly happy memories. Every other week I got to see my chemo buddy and my nurse! Both brought me comfort and joy beyond anything else those six intense chemo months! I had one of the happiest chemo sessions during my ninth trip to the Cancer Institute. We threw a surprise birthday party for my nurse. She was overwhelmed, crying like the waterhead she is, and smiling so big from joy that I thought her face was going to bust at the seams! After singing to her, exchanging hugs, and taking pictures, she cut her cake and served it to all the patients hooked up to their IV poles, kicked back in their lazy-boy chairs. After the party, I had surprise visits from friends who brought fun little gifts and told hilarious stories to keep me laughing instead of concentrating on when the red pee was coming! Even Shane surprised me by rubbing my feet and bringing lunch. Those four hours of medical imprisonment were pure joy and happiness. And if I could feel joy in having a chemo session, not sleeping at night, or having pain so deep I had to dream about Hawaii, I learned that I could certainly find it anywhere under any circumstance. I figured joy is not about what you are doing, what you own, who you are with, or remembering the better (or worse) times in life, but rather what you think about it.

Tuning In

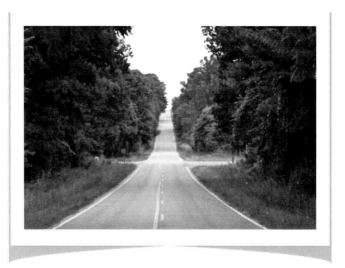

Photo by the author

Walking down a lonely highway, thinking of a
Clint Black song, and changing my state of mind.

RX: Sing.

Country music icon, Clint Black understands me. I have no musical talent whatsoever, but I certainly appreciate a good tune when I hear one! In his number one single, "State of Mind", Clint sings about walking down a deserted highway, thinking about the times when things were going the way he planned and not the way his life was actually unfolding. He thinks to himself that he has been on a lonely and bumpy road like this before, and the way he made it through was with prayer and music. He belts out, "Ain't it funny how a melody can bring back a memory. Take you to another place in time. Completely change your state of mind." Just like counseling, prayer, imagery, friends, and family are good therapy, so is music. Whether you rock it out alone or with a thousand other concert fanatics, music transports us to a deeper place and helps us to live our feelings out loud. So I say when the going gets tough, the tough not only gets going, they also get rockin'.

I was introduced to Christian artist, Aaron Keyes, and his music at a Mission Society Gathering conference. Aaron was the music worship leader. When I watched Aaron sing, gone were the lines on this man's face of worry, doubt, indecision, confusion, and fear. Instead, I saw on Aaron's face peace, praise, enthusiasm, and joy as strings of words came out of his lips. It was as if he saw God only. I think when we see an artist sing live, the music is threaded into our ears, woven into our brain, and like a sifter, is shaken and filtered purely down to the heart more so than if we just hear a song on the radio. When we hear a live artist, there is an energy, an experience, that is shared between artist and audience that is palpable and reproducible whenever we hear his songs again. That is certainly what happened for me with Aaron's music. When I needed to focus and see God only, when I was thirsty for hope and a peace-filled heart, and when I wanted to hit "replay," I had Aaron Keyes at the top of my playlist. Over and over, I was empowered by his song "Psalm 62" which says, "My soul finds rest in God alone, my rock and my salvation, a fortress strong against my foes, and I will not be shaken!"

Although many may not have heard of Aaron Keyes, most of us have heard of Ruben Studdard, known as the "Velvet Teddy Bear," the winner of season two of *American Idol.* He is an R&B artist and gospel singer, has released four albums, and is a Grammy nominee for the song "Superstar." I was fortunate enough to see him sing live in the American Idol Tour the year that he won, and his voice spoke to my heart then when he sang "Flying without Wings." It was no surprise to me then, in my deepest hours of need for strength and comfort just before my surgery, before every chemotherapy session, and as I was (and still am) being scanned in the PET scanner, that I put in my earbuds and listened to "Amazing Grace" and "Shout to the Lord" from Ruben's *I Need an Angel* CD. Just hearing Ruben sing, "I don't know why You chose me, but I'm glad You did" put courage into me for the future. Every time he sang, "Nothing compares to the promise I have in You," it was like a million coins filled up my praise bank. Yes, even in the middle of the toughest moments of life, I found a reason to sing along. The music therapy in my playlist no doubt soothed my soul when I needed it thanks to artists like Aaron and Ruben and others.

Sometimes I didn't need soothing or peace but rather I needed to be pumped up, energized, and empowered. It was then that I listened to songs like Survivor's "Eye of the Tiger." I belted along with the words "Risin' up, straight to the top, have the guts, got the glory. Went the distance, now I'm not gonna stop. Just a man and his will to survive" as I rose up to the challenge of my rival. Another artist I came to admire greatly while searching for "pump up" hits to download was Alicia Keyes who sings in "Superwoman," "I…am…a Superwoman… even when I'm a mess, I still put on a vest with an 'S' on my chest!" (How empowering is that?! Singing along with that, I could feel the cancer cells popping out of my body as I flexed my super powers!) Of course, I would be amiss if I didn't mention that Journey's "Don't Stop Believin'" was also frequently plugged into my ears. That classic deserves more than a nod when it comes to collaborating with disease fightin', times of crisis stompin', and months of hardship smackin'!

The thought of Journey's rocker guitars and long hair pulled me right into another music genre that I frequently called on during my biker chic moments like when choosing my biweekly tattoos! Sometimes I just felt like shouting, kicking something, or dancing in my living room…Oh, yes, this quiet, compliant, conservative, rule-following doctor, now the patient, can stick her tongue out and be defiant at times too! Often my ears filled with Bon Jovi's words shouting,

"We've got to hold on, ready or not. You live for the fight when it's all that you've got" in his number one hit song "Livin' on a Prayer." I spun around and danced to Adam Lambert's version of Michael Jackson's "Black or White" concentrating on the words "Now I believe in miracles, and a miracle has happened tonight!" and I did a karate kick singing, "Don't tell me you agree with me when I saw you kicking dirt in my eye."

Finally, when I was homesick and just wanted my mommy and a taste of comfort food, I rocked out to Bon Jovi's "Who Says You Can't Go Home." In doing do, I felt like I was laying my head on my rainbow pillowcase of childhood when he sang, "If it's a million miles away, or just a mile up the road, take it in, take it with you when you go." Hearing those words pumped into my ears, I easily flashed back to a different time and place, and I forgot about cancer and tests and appointments and fatigue. Instead, I remembered buying red cream soda at the local fire station with my arm in a sling in the first grade, eulogizing Mae West in front of my high school freshman English class, and the feeling of my dog, Fydeau, jumping up on my bed and licking my face when I came home from college. When I closed my eyes and lip synced along with Chris Daughtry's "Home," I also felt the love in the words, "I'm going home, back to the place where I belong. And where your love has always been enough for me." Home has many faces including where I grew up, the house where I live now, and wherever my husband, mom, dad, or brother are. The common denominators here are love, familiarity, and no doubt, somehow, a song.

Oh, Brother!

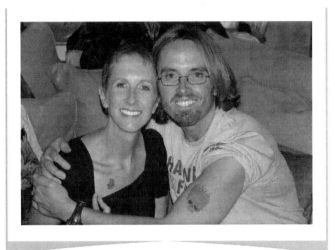

Photo by Shane Johnson

Me and my brother. For the first time ever,
his hair was longer than mine!

RX: Run a virtual marathon with
someone you love. It can be both a
grueling and a cleansing act of worship.

My brother, Eric, and I grew up in the 1970s and '80s in South Bend, Indiana. We wore plaid pants and vests that our mom made. Eric played with the original Star Wars figurines, I played with the Barbie townhouse with three levels and the plastic yellow elevator, and we both watched *The Dukes of Hazzard* and *The Love Boat*. Our parents got divorced when we were in elementary school. Mom got us. Dad moved to California. We moved down the street into a different house. Mom had a basketball hoop built on to the garage, and we thought we were the coolest kids in the neighborhood. When we were old enough to walk and feed a dog, we got one. Her name was Fydeau. She was a twenty-pound, scruffy, white mutt with a heart so big, she could wrap herself around anyone's little finger in less than ten seconds just by looking into her deep brown eyes and nuzzling her cool, velvet nose into the palm of your hand. When we were still young, one time Eric had a Putt-Putt golf birthday party. Eric, his handful of friends, Mom, and I went to try our hand at winning the coveted glow-in-the-dark hole-in-one special golf ball. We left his orange-glazed Bundt birthday cake on the dining room table. When we got back home, laughing at who made the worse golf shots, half the cake had been eaten, and Fydeau greeted us at the door, tail wagging, licking orange frosting off her chops. We loved that loyal dog, and we were loyal to each other.

Sure sometimes we got into each other's stuff and fought about typical brother and sister things, like who got the rotten end of a deal or who was smarter than the other. In the end, though, we supported each other, and the love of family outweighed our sibling rivalry. For example, one time, when I was sick on Halloween, Eric went trick-or-treating and brought back double the amount of candy that he would usually get and gave me half. When Eric and his friends were up to their teenage shenanigans, he trusted me that I wouldn't tell on him. We covered for each other and watched out for each other and for our mom.

I now live in Florida and Eric lives in Texas. He owns a sports marketing company. He loves to run, and he loves to encourage other people to run. He got me interested in running a few years ago. The difference between us is this: I run 5Ks. He runs marathons. (I guess everything really is bigger in Texas!) Nonetheless, when I was facing surgery, chemotherapy, and radiation, my brother inspired me and encouraged me to pretend that this was a marathon, and he had me laughing the whole course of the race. He did this by making up running analogies. When I couldn't run as fast or as far as I used to, he saw this speed bump on my race course as an opportunity to start over. "There are many people who would love to start over," he said. "You get to do that. You get to start over. You will be able to retrain from the start. How cool is that?" Since when does a younger brother give an older sister advice that she actually listens to? Right now, I figured, was a good time to start. He was right. In my plight, I was being handed another chance in life to start some things over.

Here are some other things I learned from my brother that helped me to run the marathon of my life.

First, it is important to train, to prepare mentally and physically for the road ahead. How did I get ready? I started running seven years before my diagnosis. I never thought I would enjoy running, but one morning I laced up my sneakers and walked out my door. The first time I hit the trail, I was only able to run a quarter of a mile. It was a start. Eventually I was running three miles at least three days a week, doing lightweight workouts, and doing sit-ups on my living room floor. Little did I know, all of that hard work and dedication was preparing me for melting away that elephant in my chest. My training ahead of time kept me physically strong enough to recover quickly from the battle that my body went through and kept me from getting too weak to walk or work. Without my baseline strength, I don't know how I could have finished the marathon of defeating cancer and feel as good as I do now.

Another thing that Eric reminded me to do was to pace myself. "When you run a race, you can't go all out in the first mile, or your will lose your steam for the miles that follow," he advised. After my surgery, Eric was there with me walking laps around the hospital hallways and then around the block at home. At the end of our block, there is a letter *S* stamped in the concrete curb. He told me to step on it. "*S* is for strength. Step on it on your walks and imagine your strength rebuilding." He was telling me that it was okay to slow down to a walking pace for the time being—but keep walking—the finish line will be there no matter how fast or slow you go. Just make sure you get there. Cross that finish line.

My brother said to eat right. Carbohydrate loading can be a good thing, but you must also eat protein and fat. He loaded our refrigerator with ground flax seeds, whey protein, stinky brussels sprouts, natural peanut butter, and organic chicken. He taught me how to make smoothies in our rickety old blender. Even my medical oncologist and radiation oncologist joined in on the running analogies. Both of them encouraged healthy eating, and they agreed with Eric. "You *are* running a marathon!" they said. They wanted me to eat a lot of calories as my body needed them to repair and build new cells—cancer-free cells. Chemotherapy and radiation treatment were burning off a lot calories and energy. They didn't want me to lose weight. The doctors wanted my "calories in" to equal if not surpass my "calories out." I took this as a free pass to eat steak and ice cream, two of my favorite foods, for breakfast, lunch, and dinner. (That didn't actually pan out by the way!)

Eric reminded me that some days I was not going to feel like running, but I needed discernment on when to exercise and when not to exercise. I knew that some days, the training would have to continue, like it or not. Some days, however, it was okay for me to take a break. Those were the days I napped on the couch or slept in late. My husband and I believed that sleep would repair me and was a natural part of the healing process. For this reason, my husband called the bed and couch my tumor annihilators. *No running today*, I told myself. *I will get back on the trail tomorrow. Today, in this bed, I have a tumor to annihilate!*

My nutty brother also said that while running a race, sometimes you will need to stop and take a crap. (Readers, if you don't like to think about poop, don't read this paragraph!) I think he was saying that even though you think you prepare before a marathon or any grueling exercise in life, sometimes you will be running along and an incredible urge to purge may come upon you. As we meander through life's trials, we need to occasionally rid ourselves of fear, anger, doubt, unhappiness, and whatever else is filling us up and slowing us down. The only way to do that is to have a cathartic moment, let our hair down, and let it all out. Letting it all out may take some straining or it may flow easy, but you cannot continue to wallow in crap. Wallowing in it, our view of life can get tainted, fuzzy even, and that can poison us. On the other hand, stopping and letting it all out is a cleansing necessity— an enema of the evils that life throws at us.

Another philosophy in the marathon advice was that during a tough run, believe it or not, there will be times when you will feel like celebrating before the race is over. Stop, relax, and have a drink when your body tells you to do so. One year, when Eric ran the Boston Marathon against freezing temperatures, rain, and a forty-mile-an-hour headwind, he knew the race was going to be tough. Eventually he saw the finish line, but he was tired and thirsty. He was only a couple of miles from the finish line when he saw a random group of friendly people at a street-side table outside of a pub flagging in runners to join them for a beer. Ready to sit for a minute and refresh, Eric saw this as an opportunity not only to celebrate his accomplishment of running the Boston Marathon, but as a way to cement a unique memory into his marathon story. So he stopped running for a few minutes, drank a beer, warmed up, dried off, and met some new friends before he continued across the finish line. I certainly don't remember Eric's time of finish in that race, but I do remember that story! I wanted stories like that! Therefore, every time I would finish a treatment, have a clear PET scan, or have a reason to celebrate some random anniversary (like one month and one day since I was cancer free) I did it.

Too often, people get stuck in a rut. We put on our blinders and walk the daily path to work, to school events, even to dinner without looking around and realizing we should celebrate that we have legs so we can walk the path, eyes so we can see our kid's basketball shot hit the rim and go in, and taste buds to savor the sweet flavor of our favorite ice cream. That's how it probably got to be our favorite in the first place, by relishing in a moment at one point in our life when we did stop running for a minute, relaxed, celebrated, and had an existential moment.

Eric also reminded me to check off the mile markers—they are mini-goals that we accomplish! When you start a race, the first mile seems to take forever, and you feel like you will never get to the finish line. Same with twelve chemotherapy sessions and twenty radiation treatments. In the middle of my marathon, some days it felt like it would never end. To stay sane, I had to check off my mile markers. *Three down, nine to go!* I said to myself. With three behind me, I was one-fourth done with chemo! When I finally finished chemotherapy, I was on the home stretch. I looked at the mile markers and landmarks I passed— surgery, mini-recovery, chemo, mini-recovery—only radiation to go! This race was almost over! For the first time, I could see the finish line.

And lastly, my brother reminded me that even when you have run twenty-six long, thirsty, and tired miles in a marathon, you have to remember that you still have two-tenths of a mile to go. Don't give up. As tired as you are and as much as you feel like puking and crawling under a bush, you are almost there. When you enter a race, you are already a winner. Just by joining, you have a goal—concentrate on marching to the finish. And then when you do, cross that line, break the ribbon, celebrate, recoup, and sign up for the next race. It is already waiting, ready or not! Catch me if you can!

You Just Might Get It All

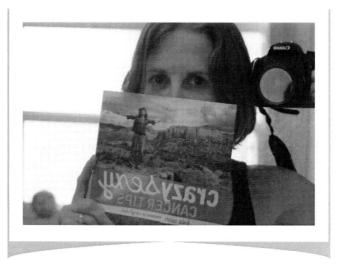

Photo by the author

A self-portrait while getting crazy, sexy
cancer tips from Kris Carr's book.

RX: Be careful what you wish for.
You just might get it all.

ix months before the lymphoma hit the fan, I was invited to tour the newest addition to Florida Hospital, the place where I spent three years completing my residency in family medicine. This new facility, the Ginsburg Tower, houses an emergency department the size of a football field as well as the Cardiovascular Institute, which includes over four hundred cardiac-care patient rooms and several state-of-the-art heart catheterization labs. When I visited, small groups of five or six of us were escorted through the well-designed ER (where there was no waiting room!) and each patient room was private and had its own TV. Then we walked up a few flights of stairs in the Ginsburg Tower to the heart cath labs, sporting million-dollar, life-saving and life-preserving equipment that we were allowed to touch! As my hands grazed the electronic controls to one of the cath tables, I believe my heart skipped a beat as I considered the gravity of the sacredness that was about to happen in these rooms in the years following its grand opening. Eventually the tour group rode the speedy elevators to the top floors of the tower, and we entered one of the high-tech patient rooms overlooking Lake Estelle. The rooms were gorgeous with dark and light-colored wood inlaid floors, big-screen televisions, private baths, and huge picture windows. Except for the standard hospital bed, it looked like a luxury hotel room! Everyone in my group was ooohing and aaahing. I remember saying out loud to no one in particular, "If I am ever sick, I want a room like this one overlooking the lake!"

Fast forward. Be careful what you wish for, you might just get it…and then some things you don't want as well. The morning after my surgery and before I was moved out of the intensive care unit, my surgeon came to see me during his rounds. He was eager to get the tubes out of my chest and bladder (thank you, God) and to get me on my feet walking the hospital hallways. I recall him saying to the nurse, "Let's get her to a step-down room and be sure to get her a nice room in the Ginsburg overlooking the lake, okay?" I smiled to myself, thinking, sure, six months ago I *wished* I could have a beautiful hospital room with caring nurses and doctors *if* I ever needed it, however, I sure didn't want to do it the way it is all happening with open chest surgery and cancer at age thirty-nine in order to get it!

Did you ever wish you had a genie in a bottle who could make your wishes come true? Ever pray for something really hard, every day, hoping God would answer your prayers? Ever dream big and think what it would be like if your dream became reality? What would you wish for, pray for, or dream about?

I am a dreamer and a doer. When the ball in Times Square dropped the year that I was going to get cancer, I made a New Year's resolution to strengthen my current friendships and to make some new friends. I wasn't sure where I would make new friends. It is difficult to meet new people when so many women my age are established in their careers, busy with their families and kids, and have a set group of friends already. I thought about joining a women's group at church, talking to other runners I saw running on the trail, or signing up for photography classes to meet people. Obviously, great places to meet like-minded people, but alas, I ended up meeting new friends in the last place I would think of meeting friends...in chemotherapy! Some fresh friendships blossomed in the chemo posse and became long-lasting, and other new friendships were only meant to be for a short time. No matter, all had their purpose in their own timing and grace.

As far as my old friends, luckily our bonds deepened and matured. I became what one friend likened to the popular Verizon phone commercial. She said, "It's like you are the guy on the phone out in the front of the pack, and there is this herd of people behind you." My Army of Angels was good to me in my selfish time of need, even when I felt like I couldn't give back as much as I received. I felt like what a queen must feel as her hive buzzes around her as they work tirelessly to make things work, to fix things, and to make things whole. I got what I wished for—friendship—but it also came with something I never expected, I had become a cancer survivor.

Another thing that I dreamed about for quite some time before my diagnosis was having some time off work. As a physician in an urgent care center, I work twelve hour days on my feet meeting the needs of patients and their families, triaging problems, reading labs and x-rays, making diagnoses, choosing treatments, giving reassurance, and balancing my time giving care, inputting notes into our electronic health records, and managing my staff. For me, although my career is fulfilling, it is tiring, and I had come to a point where I felt like I just wanted to get away for a while! Again, I made a wish, and it came true (I took about six weeks completely off), but in order to get my wish, I got some things I wouldn't wish on anyone: cancer, chemotherapy, an oncologist, a cardiothoracic surgeon, and pain.

Lastly, as a woman of faith, I longed to know God more. I was hoping for an experience or a moment that would allow me to touch the hem of His robe and to feel Him closer than I have ever felt before, then to be able to shed His light. I knew He would lead me to this moment in His timing. I don't like that I got lymphoma, but I believe that God primed me for this incredible adventure all along. I praise Him for preparing me in mind, body, and spirit and for giving me life. I realize that God is never far from me, but sometimes I am far from Him. It is me who shimmies up to (or moves away from) His side of the couch, not the other way around. During my illness, my personal relationship with God became stronger than ever as I depended on His presence twenty-four hours a day to keep me company and to give me hope, grace, humor, and a fighting spirit. Faithfully, He was there and made me sing as I went under the knife, He showed up in the form of angels at my anointing, and He kept me laughing (and eating) on my sleepless joy'roid nights! As far as shedding His light, I can only hope that these words luminesce inside of at least one other hopeful soul who dares to believe a little bit deeper and to wish for it all. I choose to believe that having lymphoma was not a test of my faith but rather a reward of my faith. I am in awe that God seems to trust me enough to challenge me to use my story as an encouragement to others and also to remain fearlessly wishing, dreaming, and praying.

Once I accepted that I was a cancer patient, that my foundation was changing, and that whenever I secretly wished for something— I might just get it all—I started to express my feelings and my needs, more openly and more maturely. I began to recognize my true emotions in a particular moment and to express myself in better ways than I had in the past. I had deepened my humanness, and I had felt it all, and in doing so, somehow I filled a void I had created in my healthy life of simply glossing over living life.

In Kris Carr's book *Crazy, Sexy Cancer Tips* Oni Faida Lampley writes,

> I don't feel wise as a result of cancer, I feel more accepting of my own humanness. And in that way I feel more connected to everybody. I'm glad there is poetry, and I'm glad there's theater, because so much of this is just life and just metaphor. Everybody's got something. You either accept it, or you fight your whole life long. Now what do you want to do? Do you want to fight against what's really happening or sink into it somehow 'cause there might be something valuable in there.

I say sink into it, dream big, wish the impossible, and keep looking up because in the end, you just might get it all.

Rachel: A Blessing

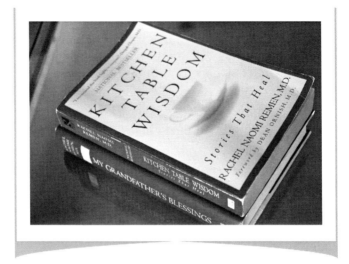

Photo by the author

Dr. Rachel Remen not only is a patient who became a doctor, she is also a mentor, an author, a healer, and a blessing to me.

RX: Count your blessings. And be one too.

an we be blessed by someone we have never laid eyes on? I believe so. I was introduced to one of my mentors twelve years before I actually met her. Her name is Dr. Rachel Naomi Remen. She is a medical physician, a master storyteller, a counselor, an author, and a spiritual teacher. She is also one of the early pioneers of the mind-body-spirit model of health. She is cofounder of the Commonweal Cancer Help Program and the founder of the Institute for the Study of Health and Illness in Bolinas, California. I was given a signed copy of her national bestseller book, *Kitchen Table Wisdom: Stories That Heal*, as a gift while I was in my second year of family practice residency at Florida Hospital in Orlando, Florida. She inscribed the book with these words: "May you find and keep the joy in our work."

When I was given this book, I was a naive, impressionable, and still-maturing young woman and physician who was seeking a mentor. As I read her stories, the following lessons are some of the concepts that poured out of her and poured into me. As I read her book, for the first time I started to understand the difference between healing and curing. Being cured implies the complete absence of disease. Being healed implies that health can be whole and vivacious even in the presence of a disease. She taught me about the life force that all living things possess. She states, "There is a tenacity toward life which is present at the intracellular level without which even the most sophisticated of medical interventions would not succeed." Reading Rachel's stories reinforced the idea that a physician's relationship with a patient and love and kindness toward a patient contributes to a patient's whole healing, sometimes even more so than a prescription. She taught me to see patients as people who have a story to tell, and not just as a diagnosis or a challenge to overcome. I have also learned from her that every person is a story and that when someone tells his or her story that is how wisdom is passed along. Rachel believes that if people think that they do not have a story to tell, they probably are not paying enough attention to life around them. We all have much to gather and to learn from each others' experiences.

Rachel tells many of her own stories in *Kitchen Table Wisdom* and in her second book, *My Grandfather's Blessings: Stories of Strength, Refuge, and Belonging.* She tells her stories from her various points of view as a granddaughter, a physician, a counselor of cancer patients, a mentor to physicians, and also as a patient herself. She is a chronic disease survivor, a warrior, who survived seven different surgeries on her abdomen to repair her ailing intestines from the time she was a vulnerable teenager. Her different roles and viewpoints along her highway in life, along with the gentle and insightful way about her, made her a wonderful mentor for me. She was to me, not just a famous person, a brilliant writer, or a popular physician, but also completely and utterly human. One other thing I learned from her was the simple concept that being human was all it took to bless another person.

As the years went by, I continued to read and reread her books. I imagined what it would be like to someday meet her, and I dreamed about the two of us sitting down in a glorious garden overlooking a California valley, drinking tea. I dreamed that she would somehow instill her wisdom, her heart, her listening ear into me through an invisible wire between us. In this vision I had, we would sit for hours, and somehow all of my experiences I once deemed "just another day" would blossom into stories worth telling. I felt like I grew to know and even love Rachel.

Finally, twelve years after being introduced to *Kitchen Table Wisdom*, I met Rachel. I was in between finishing chemotherapy and starting radiation when she traveled to Orlando to speak at a physician's summit entitled "Revitalizing the Heart of Our Work." Another mentor of mine— my counselor and friend—Dr. Herdley Paolini organized the summit. Herdley believes that in order to heal a person, you must first be a person. She understands that there is power in community, and therefore, brought hundreds of physicians and medical students together—"to gather"—for this summit.

In a big hospital auditorium (sitting by yet another mentor of mine) I gasped as Dr. Rachel Remen walked into the room. "There she is!" I whispered. She wore a salt-and-pepper casual two-piece outfit of pants and a jacket with a black silk shell underneath. She was adorned with fifty-cent-piece-sized, flat, coined-shaped silver earrings, a silver linked long chain necklace, and many unique and large, silver, artsy rings hugged her knobby fingers. Her shoes were worn in, black in color with thin laces and made of very soft leather that were almost slipper-like and bound her tiny feet tightly. It was as if her feet might burst out of them at any second! Her hair was short and white with a hint of gray, and her scalp was very pink. I almost didn't recognize her.

She looked thin, but when I saw her smile and looked at her dark, round, sparkly eyes, there was no doubt this was the Rachel of her pictures I had seen from her younger days in her books. What follows is a summary of the words and wisdom she passed on that day.

As she started to speak, she defined healing as a recovery of the heart and soul. She spoke about the power of living from the heart and becoming aware of the power that is within all of us to bless other people and the power we have to make a difference in the lives of others. In this moment of blessing, it becomes a moment of expansion and helps us remember ourselves. This ignites a spark within us. When someone sees our potential, we have an experience of self-worth. With developed self-worth, we can find meaning and purpose, and through meaning, we can transform our life experiences. Rachel said, "When we are blessed, we are led through a one way door, and there is no looking back." We can bless each other in the simple words we choose to speak, the smile we share, the eye contact we make, and the prayers we pray.

She went on to say that we are all healers of the world no matter who we are. We are here because we can make a difference. We can all be a blessing. The tools of healing are innate. Being present is simply enough. We can each be there for one another without any words ever being spoken. It is enough to believe, "I am enough. I too am human," as you bless other people. One tool of healing that Rachel spoke about was what she called generous listening. If we can do this without passing judgment, without considering if the other person is right or wrong, without the need to share our own story or viewpoint in the moment, without considering if the other person is smarter than we are, we can then really hear what is true for the other person. And if we do this generous listening, often the speaker will also hear what he or she is saying for the first time. This web of connection can only be seen through the heart as we listen and tell our stories.

Rachel went on to say,

> Our stories are like a compass. They allow us to change direction. They point toward something. They tell us what we might do, and what we might be. They make us more whole. Wholeness is human; wholeness is not perfection. Wholeness is healing. Stories can heal us.

I never thought I had a real story to tell until I was diagnosed with Hodgkin's lymphoma and lived to tell about it. I understand now that that is far from the truth. I have been alive for forty years, and I am now waking up to realize that I am the keeper of hundreds and thousands of stories in my lifetime. Many of these stories are not about me, but they are about friends and family who have simply sat down over the years at a kitchen table.

When I finally met Rachel years after our first introduction, I wished her well and thanked her for blessing me. I told her that her stories have transformed me and touched me in a thousand little ways. Reading her books again as a cancer survivor have deepened my desire and craving to live fully, love deeply, and not only count my blessings, but to be one.

Aloha Chemo

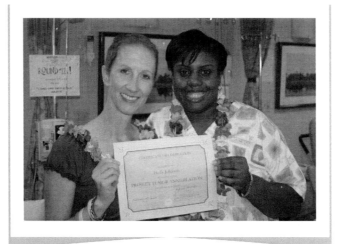

Photo by Shane Johnson

Celebrating my last day of chemo
with my angel nurse, Katina.

RX: Do what you love and love what you do.

April 1982. I was thirteen years old. Back home in Indiana it was 3:00 in the morning; I'm sure it was dark and quiet in our house on Kent Lane. The dust bunnies were settling on my rainbow-striped comforter, and the streetlight was streaming through the edges of my roll-down blinds, illuminating a triangle of light on the bright green and yellow sunflower wallpaper in my room. I, however, was a continent and an ocean away, squishing my bare feet in the warm sand. I was overlooking Diamond Head in Honolulu with my mom and brother, marveling that it was only 10:00 at night there, and I was walking on the beach! The strip of Waikiki was lit up like an airport runway, and smiling couples were walking hand in hand wearing white, fragrant leis over their necks. The spirit of aloha was palpable. I fell in love with Hawaii immediately. The young biologist in me was amazed that out of volcanic ashes, something so beautiful could rise and become so green and alive. I was promised that I would see a rainbow every day. With my head in the clouds, ever the dreamer and planner, I announced to my family, "I'm coming here for my honeymoon!"

March 1998. I was twenty-eight years old. I was sitting outdoors at the Ohana Bar and Grill of the Ka'anapali Beach Resort with my husband while watching humpback whales jump and dance in the waters between Maui, Lana'i, and Molokai. As the magnificent creatures surfaced, their tails popped up in a full fan, froze for a moment in time, winked at us, then sank into the inky blue water. My dream had come true. It was my honeymoon and I was in Hawaii.

Shane and I drove the winding road to Hana, drinking in the views of waterfalls, bamboo and sugarcane forests, pineapple farms, and black sand beaches. We also drove up the East Maui Mountains to the crater of Haleakala, passing though what looked like moon rocks, to get to the mouth of the island. Then, wearing yellow rain slickers, we biked down through the clouds, making rain as we smashed through the fog. We also walked hand in hand on the beach, smiling, wearing leis around our necks. I fell in love with Hawaii again and announced to Shane, "Let's come back here every five years!"

March 2003. I was thirty-three years old. It was almost sunset, and I was standing at the base of an active volcano in Hawaii Volcanoes National Park on The Big Island of Hawaii. We had just hiked up and then back down the side of a volcano. We walked over hardened, blackened lava rock that was so warm that it melted the tread off the bottom of our sneakers. Visible through the hardened, but porous rock, we could see molten, gooey, red lava burping forth like a blob out of the earth. The lava was intensely hot; a curious litterer threw a fast-food bag into the redness, and it burst into flames, then became a part of the ashen land. The slow-moving lava crept over the roads of the National Park, blocking our way, and moved out toward the sea. As it poured into the Pacific Ocean, it sizzled and steamed and gave the once turquoise-colored sea a dusting of new earth formation. The water near shore appeared to have a million bags of flour suspended in its watery molecules. This grayish water flowed down the shoreline, depositing itself on the black sand beach. Out of the ashes, new earth was being made…The island was expanding as if it were alive. Nothing ever stays the same.

I looked back up toward the mountain, away from the sea. The volcano was now silhouetted against an orange-pink sky. In the darkness, I could see the redness of the moving lava under the mountain's quilt along with a single file line of beaming flashlights as people walked along a path. I was astounded at the site of this spiritual mecca; it seemed as if we were all gathered in one place with one purpose—to see where we had come from. We were all marching toward something together. Out of fire and intense heat, we rose up and spewed forth, changing our shape, just like the island.

August 2008. I was thirty-eight years old. I was standing outside the Blue Ginger Cafe on the island of Lana'i eating the best egg salad sandwich I have ever had. The cafe building was a cobalt-blue color and had a wooden-framed, double-screen door that slammed shut whenever someone came in or out; I love that noise—*Creak! Bang!* The Blue Ginger Cafe was situated on the town square of downtown Lana'i City. Standing in the middle of Dole (as in the pineapple) Park looking around the square was the entire town of Lana'i City: the library, the community center, the school, the grocery store, two restaurants, the gym, a jewelry store, a shop selling wind chimes, and the post office. People were coming and going out of the shops, and kids were chasing each other down the sidewalk after class. With mayo and hard-boiled eggs dripping down my chin, I fell in love with the quaintness of the town and its fervor for small-town island life. I couldn't believe that I was standing in Hawaii for the fourth time in my life—my fourth aloha island! I was content and happy and completely oblivious that the next time I would close my eyes and "visit" our fiftieth state, it would be under completely different circumstances.

November 2009. I was thirty-nine years old. I was sitting in my brown, lazy-boy chair as the last dose of ABVD was coursing through my veins. My feet may have been planted in Orlando, Florida, but my soul was in my true love locale, Maui. For my final round of chemotherapy, I brought Hawaii to the Cancer Institute. Friends, family, and other patients were each given a Hawaiian lei to wear. I brought photo albums from our Hawaii trips to keep my eye on the prize—paradise— no more of this beaten road called cancer. I set up a mini beach scene at my chair-side table complete with sand, a chaise lounge, shells, an umbrella, and flip-flops. I sat back with the IV tube coming out of my chest and listened to my favorite luau songs from the islands from a CD that we had bought on our honeymoon. In the aloha spirit, many friends came to visit me on my last day in that chair as I completed Project Tumor Annihilation. We served pineapple slices and cake. Out of a deep well called cancer, I was growing, rising out of the ashes, burning off the residue, and making new earth, new cells.

My oncologist came by and said that he didn't know what they would do without me in my chair. He told me that they would miss me. I was humbled and grateful to think that I had come this far with a little grace, a sense of humor, an example of how to share a load, and with my life. And now, no more chemo, no more four to five hour appointments sitting in the brown recliner, no more two week cycles of beatings, no more red pee, no more Neulasta! I went home and had an egg salad sandwich and imagined slamming the screen door on chemo. Then, on my last Neulasta Friday, I wore my cowgirl hat, and the Cancer Institute staff and I all lined danced to Debbie Harry's "I Will Survive"! It was time to hula, and it was time to reclaim myself…But first, aloha to chemo and hello to radiation.

I'm Toast

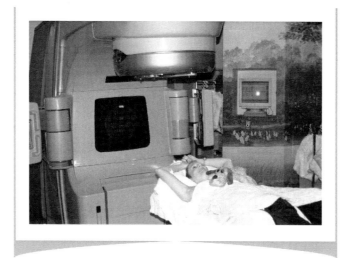

Photo by Shane Johnson

The Star Wars–like radiation treatment table with its big blue arm circling around me and Biscuit.

RX: To get through the muck, you may have to coach your mind through a paradigm shift in order to heal.

How do you like your toast? I like mine lightly browned and evenly crunchy with no burnt edges. How do we make toast? A toaster works by changing electrical energy into heat energy. The heat, or infrared radiation, radiates from the loops of the glowing orange metal coils inside of the toaster. If there is not enough radiation, you won't get the desired results. If there is too much radiation, well, you have just burned the toast!

When I met the radiation oncologist for the first time, he bluntly stated that although the chemotherapy got rid of my visible tumor, it was radiation that would be the cure. Medical radiation works much differently than a toaster, but it certainly can still make you feel like toast! It is a mysterious science that works at a cellular level to destroy fast-growing cells, like cancer cells. It hurts some normal cells as well, but normal cells recover quickly, whereas cancer cells do not. Under guided radiation treatment, cancer cells bite the dust, and noncancerous, normal healthy cells grow back and thrive. Therefore, medicinal radiation energy would, in essence, be my life-saving treatment. This was a profound reality to me: I was undergoing life-saving treatments. Until this time I hadn't really thought of that in such a pure, true way until I was about to start this next phase. In *Kitchen Table Wisdom* Dr. Rachel Remen states that "survival in a setting of life-threatening illness may involve a willingness to let go of everything but life itself." Life: living life, committing to life, choosing life. Life is more than just being alive—it is loving, serving, finding joy, paying attention, living intentionally, feeling it all.

Radiation treatment was a big commitment. I had to go every day, Monday through Friday, for twenty treatments. Every weekday, I entered the cozy waiting room filled with wicker furniture with tropical fabric seat cushions, and I used a card with a barcode on it to "check in." This signaled my radiation technicians that I was there and ready for treatment. I smiled at the other people in the waiting room and often grabbed a packet of graham crackers or cookies to snack on while waiting. When my name was called, I was led down a cheery garden and country-themed painted mural hallway to the changing rooms. I then had to undress and put on the same blue hospital gown that I wore when I had surgery.

Using more guided imagery, I brought "invisible powers" with me in a couple of tokens that I would clasp in each hand. In one hand, I held a huge nutmeg-colored acorn that I had found on a walk at the foot of a towering oak tree. I too wanted to burst into a mighty oak! I had my family symbolically instill several acorns with the fruits of the spirit: love, joy, peace, patience, kindness, goodness, gentleness, faithfulness, and self-control at our Thanksgiving dinner. Except for the one I held in my hand every day during radiation treatments, I gave away all the acorns to my chemo posse and to other friends. I hoped that the seeds would mean something to someone else and that it would bring blessings to their beholders too. In the other hand, I held a verse from Zephaniah 3:17: "The

Lord your God is in your midst, a mighty one that will save; he will rejoice over you with gladness; he will quiet you by his love; he will exult over you with loud singing!"

I walked into the radiation room where the cold blue Star Wars–looking Trilogy machine loomed behind a one-foot-thick lead wall and door. I lay supine on the hard table on top of a sheet; my knees were propped up by a triangular shaped pillow. My head and arms rested above my head in a custom, made-for-me, hardened mold of my upper body, arms, head, and neck. I felt the technicians pull me from side to side with the sheet as they lined me up on the table. They used three permanent tattoos that they placed on my chest to line me up with the beams. (I asked for tattoos of Maui, Oahu, and The Big Island, but they told me that they didn't have their Hawaiian island stencils with them the day they were needled under my skin, and I had to settle for gray-blue dots! (Drats! Foiled again!)

On the table, lined up in the plastic mold of me, I looked straight up into the jaws of the machine and saw a white light that was shaped like a line of Frankenstein sutures, a grid of sorts, that must line up with my spine, my midline. Then I was left alone with my thoughts, my acorn, my power verse, the Trilogy machine, and some overhead music. The lead door and curtain closed and the door sealed shut. (*I am safe in the event of a nuclear attack*, I think to myself!)

I closed my eyes and felt the talisman in each hand. The whirring of the CT scan was a buzz in my ears as its panels flanked me, and they took a quick picture to make sure that I was still and centered for the beam. I was frozen in that galactic pose for seven minutes. *See God only and feel the fruits of the Spirit around you,* I told myself. The Trilogy arm, a big periwinkle-blue circular disc circled around to my back. I heard the crackle of the teeth of the machine moving, then the buzz of the radiation, and I saw the white sign with the red letters, "beam on," light up. I was still as the oval arm circled around me, zapping me with millions of kilovolts twice at each of seven different angles. When the machine was directly overhead, I looked up into the glass belly of the monster. It was a rectangle shape, and inside of it were dark silver, drill-bit-like teeth, hundreds of them, staring down at me with their fangs. They shifted and moved, opening some gaps in its wicked smile, closing some others. The final opening pattern of these drill-bit teeth was a special shape, designed just for me, I now remembered. *Wait a minute,* I thought. This machine wasn't a foe. It was saving my life and protecting me from recurrence. Trilogy was no longer menacing jaws. It was the eye of healing, and I was staring straight into it.

The buzz of the radiation filled my ears for a few more minutes, and then I was done. As the technicians reentered the room, I slowly moved to get up. It was hard to sit up. I felt liked burnt toast, like I had swallowed the sun, and it was now radiating outward. I was warm from the inside out. My chest ached. It felt like someone was encircling my ribs in a big bear hug. At the same time,

I felt like I was going to explode, like I was enlarging. I eventually reversed my steps down the garden hallway, to the changing room, back out to the waiting room, and off to the mall; I had a bigger bra to go buy!

Birthday Gift

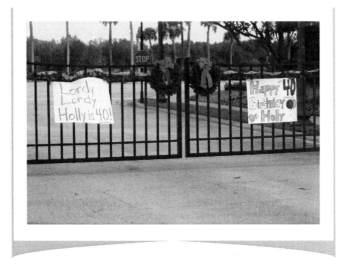

Photo by the author

This is what I woke up to on December 16
before my twelfth radiation treatment.

RX: Embrace your birthday. It is a blessing, not
a curse to grow older. Birthdays aren't for wimps.

It was a cool December morning, and I was lying in bed under the comfortable covers. I heard the front door gently click shut as my husband pulled on the door handle to ensure the door was secure and locked. I heard his Honda Civic start up and drive away. I stretched out and then drifted back to sleep, moments later to be awoken with the sound of the front door opening. As Shane walked back into the house and then the bedroom, I said, "Did you forget something?"

He said, "No, you need to get out of bed and come see something."

Begrudgingly leaving the warmth of the bed, slipping into a sweatshirt and fluffy slippers, I followed him out to the car. "Where are we going?" I asked.

He replied, "You'll see. Just get in the car."

He drove me out to the front gates of our subdivision. There, plastered for the neighborhood to see were two large white poster boards with big bright letters exclaiming, "Lordy, Lordy, Holly is 40!" and "Happy Birthday, Dr. Holly!" I loved it and started laughing, my now cold pj's shaking and hitting against my skin. My sneaky friends had come over late at night to hang the signs, while neighbors tooted their horns and shouted, "Yeah!" out their car windows at them as they prepped for the surprise. When I saw the signs in the morning light, Shane asked me if I wanted to take them down. I said, "No way! I want those up there all day long!" I was elated to get old rather than to not make it to my next birthday!

After Shane took me back home, I crawled into bed hoping for a few more hours of sandman time until I had to get ready to go to the hospital for my twelfth radiation treatment. Then, the doorbell rang, so I was out of bed for the second time way too early on my birthday morning. It was a flower delivery for me—two dozen beautiful, perfect roses of all colors from my work family! I was leaping out of my skin, and I hadn't even been toasted yet with radioactive beams that day! I succumbed to not getting any more sleep, showered up, and trudged onward to the hospital. When I got to the threshold of the Star Wars room, the door was shut. Eventually, one of the technicians beckoned to me for my turn on the table. I wasn't prepared for what happened next!

I stepped on the other side of the thick, lead door. A group of techs jumped out at me and yelled, "Happy Birthday!" and took pictures of my totally surprised face and thinly hair-crowned head! There were birthday balloons and ribbons all over the room. I started jumping up and down; I was so excited and touched that they remembered my special day and went out of their way to make December 16th's treatment so memorable for me!

Later in the day, my sneaky friend, Nancy (who made the Lordy, Lordy signs) came over to bring me a birthday present. She called ahead of time to make sure that I was home. (Of course I was home—fried and exhausted from the cumulative effects of twelve radiation treatments!) When she rang the doorbell, she was standing on my front step holding her clinging three-year-old in her arms. She asked, "Can you come out to my car to get your gift? Slade won't let me put him down."

I gave a willing, "Yes, certainly!"

As I walked out of the front door and turned right to face the driveway, oh my goodness, there was another surprise! My mom, who lives four states away, was standing there with her arms out, face beaming, saying, "Happy Birthday!" I started jumping up and down for the second time that day, laughing, landing in my mom's arms, then crying, blubbering out, "Mom, thank you so much for having me!" Well, then my mom started crying, then Nancy was crying, and poor little Slade was probably just thinking to himself, *Why are all these women crying?*

For my fortieth birthday finale, I planned for my family, some close friends, my chemo buddy and chemo nurse and their families to come to dinner to help me celebrate turning a milestone birthday, laced with a new decade and being cancer free. In my heart I knew that I would rather be forty and cancer-free than thirty-nine and have Hodgkin's lymphoma again! We gorged ourselves through piles of delicious Italian pastas and tiramisu. For me, it was a perfect and wonderful birthday, and I couldn't have asked for a better gift!

I have always been one to embrace my age and celebrate my birthday in good spirits and with gusto, but let me tell you, I will never look at birthdays quite the same ever again! Our birthdays are a gift, an absolute gift, and it is a privilege to live each year of my life and to share those years with family, friends, colleagues, patients, and even strangers I smile at on the street or sit next to on an airplane. It is an honor to just be present. Through our presence, we are all a gift.

My Redhead Moments

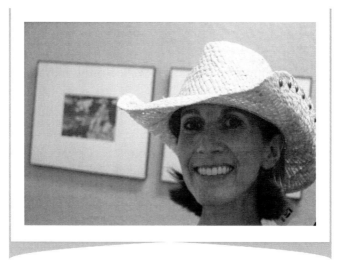

Photo by the author

I have nothing but good moments
when I wear my cowgirl hat.

RX: Cowboy up. Reclaim yourself.

P eople say that redheads have a temper. I am not sure where that idea originated; however, I do not think that I am one of them. For validation, I questioned my mother about it once. I asked, "Mom, did I have a stereotypical redhead temper when I was growing up?"

She laughed and replied, "Well, I think maybe you slammed your door once."

It must be my nature because, apparently, I am not as fiery as my hair stereotypes me to be. However, amid my usual positive and upbeat mind-set, creative energy, and deep faith, I still have had a bad day or two in my life. In fact, the year of my cancer, when I was feeling it all, I had my share of having what I labeled as "reality moments," including a temperamental redhead one!

Just four days after my second round of chemotherapy, I remember waking up and feeling really angry. It was incredulous to me that I had Hodgkin's lymphoma! I was upset that I had pain every morning and that I had to take medication to get relief. I was annoyed that every morning it felt like my lower intestines were in a blender! I was angry that my life felt like it was upside down. I was upset that this wasn't a dream. I was grieving that I had to have surgery and my body didn't look the same as before! I hated that I couldn't run. I hated that I was consumed by thoughts of my diagnosis. On top of that, I didn't want to go back to work! I was having a reality moment, and I was furious about it! This mood wasn't typical for me, red hair or next-to-no hair! For my own sanity, I had to snap out of it! I found an orange mini-nerf basketball and started kicking it around the house. *Bam!* It hit the wall, and it felt good. *Bam!* It hit the front door and bounced back at me, and it felt even better. My husband and I made a game out of it, and we kicked that ball back and forth for hours along our long entryway. It was a fun and (a usually) injury-free way to let off some steam.

After I kicked off my bad mood, my third chemotherapy session rolled around; I didn't want to go. At that point, I still had ten more doses to look forward to, so it was a little early in the game to be tired of going to treatments already, but that was simply how I felt in that moment. I wanted my cancer to go away and for my treatments to end, so I could put the whole experience behind me. The reality at that moment, however, was that it was not over. There were many months ahead of me before I would be well again. Every time I got poked at my port site and watched the red Jesus juice flow through the IV and into me, I was slapped with a reality moment—I had cancer. The less joyful emotional moments like this were mixed with the excitement and celebration of finishing each treatment. I often felt like this really could not be happening to me. *I must be living someone else's life,* I would think to myself. Then, I would feel a craving for a Taco Bell bean burrito or the start of a hot flash; I would taste the terrible bluck in my mouth or look in the mirror at my short, thinning hair, and I would remember...*This is real. This* is *happening to me. This is not a dream. I am surviving and fighting cancer, trying to go on living, to have my normal life back. Who was I? Where did normal go?*

Normally, I had a fairly monotonous life scheduled around home and work. As I mentioned, I am a physician. I work ten and twelve-hour shifts in an urgent care clinic. I help people when they have ear pain or a cough, if they cut their finger and they need stitches, or when they twist their ankle while skateboarding and need a splint and crutches. Then, on my days off, I have my routine. I enjoy watching the morning talk show banter. Then I usually tie up my laces, put on a baseball cap, and hit the pavement to run, walk, or bike. After pumping my muscles, I shower, run errands, clean house, meet with friends, or spend time with my husband. I attend church on the weekends. I call my mother once or twice a week. Living this life, I felt balanced and healthy in every way.

Hit from the blindside, however, all my normal went away. I couldn't work full time anymore. I was eventually too tired to run. It was hard to keep the house clean. I had to nap every day. I had to visit my oncologist once a week. My doctor told me that I would arrange my treatments around my normal schedule. Baaa-loney! Most parts of my new normal life were instead arranged around those treatments and how I felt after them. My temporary new life was anything but boring, but it certainly did not feel remotely close to normal. After seven months of getting beat up with treatments, I couldn't even breathe like I used to!

Normally our breathing is an unconscious bodily function given to us by God to cleanse ourselves; we breathe in air and oxygen to feed our cells, and we exhale our carbon dioxide waste. We don't think about it, yet at least ten to twelve times a minute, we live on because we breathe! After my eleventh radiation treatment, it started to get hard to breathe and hard to swallow. I burped from the depths of inside of me that felt like I would split open. My cilia were paralyzed, and I coughed more in order to sweep out the dust. It hurt to inhale, and it became impossible to exhale.

Ultimately, I had to master how to breathe again. I had to go deep inside of me, "cowgirl up," eliminate negativity, and put on my warrior paint. Only I could do this for my redheaded self. I remembered what normal felt like, and I wanted it back! I wanted to run, to lift a gallon of milk without needing to use two hands, to lie down without pain, to swallow without the ball in my throat, and to run my fingers through my long hair. In my quest for normalcy in the year of the fog, I discovered that learning to breathe again wasn't just a physical thing, but a mental, emotional, and spiritual one as well. To get well, I had to breathe more effectively from a deeper place. I had to get rid of inflammation—things that were upsetting the balance of my own homeostasis. I learned that each moment in life was a fleeting breath, often a sigh too brief to measure. I learned to set boundaries for myself and to set my own pace. I forgot about the person in front of me and the person behind me telling me what I should do or should not do. I learned to rest better, sleep deeper, and dream bigger. Before cancer, I didn't necessarily know what I needed or wanted in any given moment, but I do now. I promised myself that I would continue to participate in this life, so I didn't miss my life. Through it all, I did "cowgirl up," and I found that during this incredible adventure, I was reclaiming myself. Hmmm…as a matter of fact, through it all, maybe I was more "normal" than ever.

I'm Gonna Blow

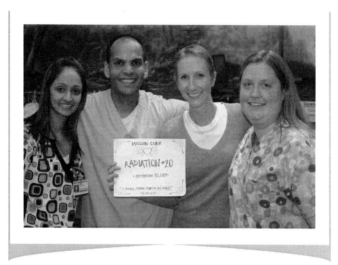

Photo by Shane Johnson

My radiation team, Angie, Shay, and Angel, and
me on my last day of radiation treatment.

RX: Be prepared. The direction and speed of the wind
can change in a heartbeat. Even the strong may
become weak, and the weak may become strong.

If the bulb of a blood pressure cuff could cough, I know what it would feel like. The black rubbery sphygmomanometer head would be in the clutches of a puffy, liver-spotted nurse's hand. She would tease it at first, a slow squeeze, then release, followed by another squeeze, and another until the frenzied pace began: squeeze, squeeze, squeeze, cough, cough, cough—like the fit of a wound-up three-year-old not getting his way.

I felt like I was losing my mind. I didn't expect this. Granted, I didn't expect the Central Florida winter twenty-six degree temperature would poke its chilly fingertips into my alveoli either. I felt miserable. I had breezed through my treatments so far, so why this? Why now? My cough had resurfaced to the point of giving me severe enough rib pain that I had to splint myself, hugging my arms underneath my right breast and side. The cough was dry and uncomfortable, and cold weather and any scent would set it off. I inhaled and then I felt like I couldn't exhale all the air that I breathed in. I literally couldn't get air out of me! I felt like I was gonna blow up! Even my bra felt too tight wrapped around my chest. It felt like I was clutched in a constant bear hug from a sumo wrestler. I became exhausted physically and mentally. I wanted to crawl in a hole and curl up in a ball…Only I couldn't curl up; it hurt too much!

I called my medical oncologist, and he told me to come see him. Frustrated, but patiently, I waited in his office before he was able to work me in between his other patients. My normal vital signs were taken and my clear lungs were auscultated. As I hacked and coughed and splinted my ribs, exasperation was written all over my face. The physician ordered a stat chest CT scan. It seemed like a waste to me, but I reminded myself that I was the patient, not the doctor in this situation. Although I suggested the possibility of more medications, time, and waiting for the weather to warm up, I was shot down, and therefore, I yielded.

My husband and I traipsed to the hospital radiology department. An IV was started in my left arm. I was cold. I was crying. I didn't want to have the procedure. I was coughing like I had a chicken bone stuck in my throat. I slid into the scanner, a circle of energy whirring around me—here I go again—breathe, hold your breath, breathe. Suddenly I felt flushed and warm in my arm, my chest and my bladder (finally for the first time that day, I was warm!) and I got a metallic taste in my mouth. Then, it was over in a matter of less than ten minutes. The IV was out, and I was dismissed. Only, I had too much pain in my ribs to even sit up on my own! I didn't know whether I wanted to laugh or cry. I had to ask for help.

As Shane and I started the long trek back to the Cancer Institute, I was tired and weak. I couldn't breathe. I sat down, defeated. Then, I really lost it! I was sobbing, I was coughing, my ribs were killing me; mucous was flowing out of my nose—and I didn't care—and tears were streaming over my cheeks in to my lap. I couldn't pull myself together. I sat in the Florida Hospital chapel, rocking back and forth trying to soothe myself when suddenly in my head, I heard my church's worship team singing, "For the Lord is good. And his mercies will not fail us. They are new each day..." *Have mercy on me today, Lord*, I started to pray. My strength restored for the moment, we stood up and walked slowly out of the hospital.

Eventually we made it to the car, and there, I lost it again! This time it was a big cry with big tears, and at this point, I didn't even want to pull myself together. With Kleenex stuffed up my nose and my head against the steering wheel, I cried until I was too tired to cry anymore. "This stinks!" I wailed over and over until I finally realized that I just wanted to go home.

This was definitely one of the most difficult times for me emotionally and physically. Less than a year ago I was running three days a week and pumping out hundreds of sit-ups a week. Now I was referred to my fourth specialist within nine months! This time, I had an appointment with a pulmonologist, a lung specialist. He told me that the CT showed three cracked ribs— aha, that's what hurt so much!—but that the lungs looked normal. However, I had follow up lung function testing in his office that showed some abnormalities and proved that I couldn't get the air out of me! He diagnosed me with reversible interstitial pneumonitis. It was due to the combination of the radiation treatment and the bleomycin chemotherapy medication (the bananas!). As a result, my lungs were hypersensitive, and I was coughing like the life was being squeezed out of me. At this point, I just wanted "normal" back...But what was normal anymore?

Celebration of Life

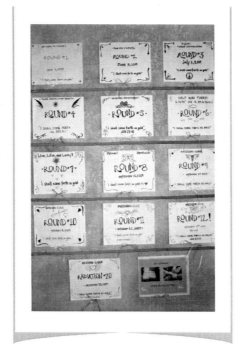

Photo by the author

The wall that saved me.

RX: Throw a party.

I am a survivor. From the moment I was born, to the moment I was diagnosed with Hodgkin's lymphoma, to this day, I have been a survivor. On a cold February morning I stood in the shower as my cancer mantra (from Job 23:10) flooded over me: "But He knows the way I take; when he has tested me, I will come forth as gold." Standing with the hot water raining down on me, I was awash with raw emotion and lathering down with surgical soap. My heart and mind were focused on what was about to happen. In just a couple of hours, my port was coming out.

The night before, I lay in bed wide awake from nerves and a six week prednisone high (the treatment for my lungs so I didn't blow!) and I palpated my Power Port for the last time. I could feel the lump under my skin: it felt like a hard triangle and was slightly movable. Inside the triangle, I felt the three pinpoint dots that were used as landmarks for accessing the port. When I twisted my torso just so, I could actually see one of the dots roll under my skin. These three landmarks were also set in a triangular shape, and at the center, I felt a hard, rubbery area (with a little less give than the body of the port itself) where my nurse would expertly insert the port needle. Then I ran my fingers over the catheter of the Power Port, which I could also easily see rise up underneath my skin if I twisted my torso just so. It was a hard, plastic tube that came up out of the body of the port and turned toward the right before disappearing under my bony clavicle and entered my subclavian vein. Invisibly it snaked its way into the right upper chamber of my heart. I rolled onto my stomach and felt the familiar tug of the port under my skin, chest, and collarbone. Now, standing in the shower, I wondered if I would ever miss that sensation. (My answer…probably not!)

As the hot water rushed over me and the unique smell of the chlorhexidine soap mingled with the steam, a second thought came to me. I remembered back in May when the port was put in, I had thought to myself, *What I would feel like on this day, the day it was coming out?* All summer, fall, and winter I thought that I would have to leave the port in for six to twelve months after my treatments before my oncologist would want it out. Therefore, I was surprised that he allowed me to remove it in less than two months after finishing treatments! I felt joyful, gleeful, and grateful as the significance of this milestone—surviving and defeating cancer—rang loudly with the removal of the port. What I didn't anticipate feeling back in May, when this day came, however, was this strange feeling of transition and confusion. This was going to be an identity shift for me as the port came out. Like the shower washing off dirt and sweat, I was washing off some stuff I just didn't need anymore…or did I? I was moving from being a cancer patient back to just me. Would I just disappear into the background of life and go back to living life as I knew it before cancer? What were my responsibilities as a survivor? Did I even have any?

To help make that transition, I had a "Celebration of Life" party and filled our home with family and friends to celebrate how our lives were uniquely all woven together. I wanted the party to feel warm and cozy, like a home cooked meal making my belly full and my lips smiling and saying, "Mmm…mmm…This is good!" Therefore, five days after my port (but not the power!) removal loved ones poured through our door—over forty of them! My eyes wide open, blinking with tears, my grateful heart was pounding as our home overflowed with the blessing of a support system like this.

I felt like I had to say something. I stood in front of one of the light golden-brown textured walls in our house where I had hung all of my chemo and radiation signs. There they were: splayed one after another, mile marker after mile marker, a visual cue of the marathon I had run. As I hung them one at a time that morning, I eventually stepped back and saw the big picture. Suddenly, it was like I had spent hours of focusing closely and intensely on an ugly but tolerable bug in front of me, and I had stepped back and now saw a beautiful autumn forest and gorgeous sun rays speckling golden leaves. Wow! I was overcome with feelings of sadness, gladness, and awe that I had been diagnosed with cancer, endured major chest surgery and an ICU stay, been intravenously dripped and dosed with twelve chemotherapy treatments—forty-eight different doses of these drugs—endured PET scans every two months, and been buzzed with twenty radiation doses. As of July I was cancer free. As of February 15 the following year, I was port free, and as of February 20 I was celebrating life, celebrating a new season, celebrating surviving.

The children at the party sat at my feet, and the adults stood and sat around, all eyes on me. I was nervous as I shared with them the story of Biscuit and how the caramel-colored, funny-looking stuffed dog came to live with me because a little boy chose him for me with hope that my boo-boo would heal. I admitted to everyone that Biscuit did make me feel better because of the love in which he was shared. After returning Biscuit to its owner, I felt like I still needed to say more. This is what I shared: Just as the Lord's Prayer states, "Thy kingdom come, thy will be done *on earth* as it is in heaven," we are here on this planet to build heavenly families. This room is full of heaven on earth for me. You all are my family. Luke 34:11 says, "For where you store your treasure, there will be your heart also." These eyes looking at me in this room are where I store my treasures—you are my own heart walking around outside of my body. I *could* have fought cancer without you, but I certainly would not have *wanted* to. Thank you for being here, for praying for me, for loving me, and for helping me to live strong and be a survivor.

I loved having the house packed with people coming and going, bringing food, eating, hugging one another, kids playing, and lots of smiling and laughing. I loved that one of my three-year-old friends fell asleep on the couch and that one of the other kids sat on him, and he didn't wake up! I loved that the three-month-old baby in the bunch slept in the middle of our big bed for a nap. I loved that friends were mingling and that as the party wound down, my mom, mother-in-law, sister-in-law, and other women cleaned the kitchen. I loved that some friends stayed late and talked with our families as it grew dark. I love my friends and my family. I love life. I love my life. I love that the celebration doesn't end here.

Docere, Studium, Pati

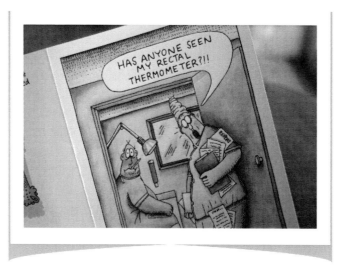

Photo by the author

The front of a get-well card I received as
a patient that makes me laugh.

RX: Learn from others.

I learned from one of my nurses that the word *doctor* was derived from the Latin word *docere*, meaning "to teach." I agree. As a physician, it is my duty to teach patients about how to live their best healthy life. When they are afflicted with illness or injury, I teach them about their diagnosis; and I present them with the options, risks, benefits, and side effects of different treatments. I also consider their whole health as I consult with them, and maybe even pray with them, thus, teaching them about the ultimate Healer.

The etymology of the word *student* comes from the Latin word *studium*, meaning "study or application," originally "eagerness." As any teacher (or doctor) will tell you, a teacher is really an eternal student, passionate about learning new information or deepening the knowledge that he already has.

Finally, the word *patient* comes from the Latin verb *pati* meaning "suffering." Doctors may tell you that they are diligent students, but our culture tells us that doctors make the worst patients. I don't think that has to be true. If doctors study, learn, and implement healthy behaviors from our own patients, like being honest, being strong, and being patient, we can become the best of patients when our turn comes. And it will come.

Mrs. Turner was lying flat on her back on the exam table, her feet up in stirrups. She was a seventy-something, feisty, skinny, black woman with a rich history of growing up in rural Eatonville, Florida, with thirteen grandchildren and a patch of collard greens between the palmettos in her backyard. She was missing most of her teeth, and when she talked, her sausage-shaped tongue slithered in and out of the space where her front teeth should have been. Her gums were a purplish color, her frizzy black hair was spattered with white, frizzier hairs, and she didn't wear a speck of makeup. She was the real deal. She grinned up at me from the table. It was my second year of family medicine residency, and she had come to see me for her annual well-woman exam. I seated myself on the short, spinning stool at her feet and asked my nurse to pass the speculum so I could begin the exam. I started to pull back the sheet that was covering Mrs. Turner's lower half when she raised up a brown skeletal hand with neatly trimmed nails. I couldn't imagine what she was about to do or say when she opened her toothless mouth and exclaimed, "Wait a minute, Dr. Johnson! I'm gonna blooooow!" I felt a slow curl of a grin start to form on the side of my lips as I pulled the sheet back over her. I stepped back, made eye contact with my nurse, and then howled with laughter along with my patient as she passed a loud and long gaseous fart. In that completely naked moment, I learned the importance of patients' honesty with me, even in their most embarrassing moments. If she hadn't been truth bearing in that moment, I would certainly have had an unexpected (and stinky) surprise square in my face that day! When I thought about her bluntness and honesty, I thought to myself, *If I am ever a patient, I would like to be like Mrs. Turner: honest, open, and in the process, even a little funny.*

Although I learned in my second year of residency that being an honest patient was important to being a healthy patient, it was during my third year that I started to learn about the inherent strength of a human being. An intern and I were called to a code blue, a devastating moment when a patient in the hospital stops breathing and his heart stops beating. We ran through the halls and took the fastest elevator we could find; our long white doctors' coattails were flying out behind us. When we arrived in the ICU code room, the nurses were already frantically giving chest compressions, manually bagging Mr. Finch to help him breathe, and pushing medications like lidocaine and epinephrine into IVs. The room looked like a tornado had hit: commands were being shouted, there were empty saline bags and plastic needle caps and sleeves all over the floor, and there was a defibrillator hooked up to the patient with a horrible-looking flatline on the electrocardiogram. There must have been ten or twelve staff members hovered around the patient's bed. We pumped and pushed and squeezed and shocked the patient for thirty minutes with no return of spontaneous breathing or heartbeats. The patient was dead. The code was called off. The intern had the unenviable job of treading to the waiting room where the patient's family was pacing back and forth on the well-worn carpet. It suddenly seemed very dark and heavy in the hallways as if the sun had stopped streaming through the windows. I followed the intern and watched as he approached the family, said something quietly, and embraced them. As I watched this incredibly sad, inevitable human experience, a nurse showed up at my side, and whispered, "Dr. Johnson, Mr. Finch is breathing." I interrupted the intern and explained to the family that we would be right back. We calmly walked back into the room we had just left and watched the chest of the patient rise and fall for his last breath on this side of heaven. Finally, the room seemed to light up again, all was quiet, and a peace hovered over the room. I stood there in awe of the moment and the strength it takes for a human to endure a lifetime, to flatline, then to return in order to inhale and exhale the few last breaths in front of witnesses—two lowly residents. We were both wondering, if we were ever in a crisis like Mr. Finch, if we could be that strong to come back from the dead if even for an instant.

Although during my training I responded to many code blues, rarely does anyone survive. When a code blue is called, the patient is already clinically dead. The first time you actually save a life, and you bring someone back from the dead, you never forget it. Long after residency, I was working in an urgent care center seeing the usual ear infections, sore throats, sprained ankles, and sunburns when someone yelled, "Doctor, come outside!" I burst through the door to the waiting room and saw a man lying on the sidewalk in front of our clinic, his face as purple as a plum, and his chest heaving. He was not moving his arms or legs and was not responding as his friend stood over him, reciting his name, "Dan! Get up, Dan!" Apparently, he had pulled up in his white Ford 250 pickup truck outside of our front doors, opened his car door, and fell out onto the ground, smack on his back. He was wearing blue jeans, a red flannel button-down shirt, and brown work boots. I quickly felt for a pulse…thready. He was having agonal respirations and clearly was going to die on our concrete threshold if we didn't do something fast. I stacked one of my hands on top of the other and started pumping on his chest while a staff member put a medical bag ventilator to his mouth and started assisting him with his breathing. We put a defibrillator on the patient's bare chest as I talked to him, "Dan, stay with us! We are here to help you! We are going to shock your heart now!" We all said, "I'm clear! You're clear! Everybody's clear!" just as we learned in basic life support class, and we shocked the patient. No response. We shocked him again and…his heart beat came back! After that, the paramedics arrived, took over his care, and transported him to the emergency room. He was airlifted to the best heart hospital in Orlando, had an emergency triple heart bypass, and the next morning was sitting up in his hospital bed eating breakfast! The strength of the human will to live cannot be underestimated. It is woven into our being to be strong, to live strong, to stay strong if we just call on it and breathe into it. After I learned that this patient went from one day barely breathing, flat as a pancake outside our front door, to the next day, sitting up in bed eating pancakes, I thought to myself, *If I am ever in a life-threatening situation, I would like to believe that I can be strong and live strong enough to breathe another day, just like Dan.*

One last lesson I learned from a patient was to be patient. Going to a doctor's appointment is never like buzzing through a drive-thru, giving an order, and getting instant gratification of salty fries and a milkshake. I wonder, is that why we started calling patients, patients? Not because they were suffering but rather because they had to be (patient, that is)? One afternoon, I was three hours behind schedule in the walk-in center when I breezed into an exam room and met Jason, a guy with a sore throat and cough. I shook his hand and apologized profusely for his wait. I even told him that I hated to wait myself! He looked me in the eye, and he didn't interrupt me as I explained how I could only see one patient at a time and how crazy busy we were on that particular day. I listened to his reason for coming in, examined him, and came up with a treatment plan. He thanked me for helping him, and as I contemplated his incredibly thankful and calm demeanor, I asked him how he became such a patient man. He then told me that he was a melanoma cancer survivor. He often had to sit and wait for hours to get his treatments and to see his busy oncologist. He said that his life depended on him being patient, and if he hadn't been, his life wouldn't have been saved in quite the same way. He said,

> Being patient helped me to survive. I had no choice but to be patient. Besides, a doctor can't work under all that pressure to be on time all the time. Emergencies happen. Life happens. And if you are in too much of a hurry and you are not patient, you just might miss the point.

Yes, I thought to myself. *I often hear what patients are really trying to say long after I have examined their ears, wrapped up their ankles, and written their prescriptions.* I also thought to myself, *If I am ever a patient, I would like to be just like Jason: patient, even in my suffering.*

Honesty, sense of humor, strength, and patience are virtues that I admire. I watched as my healthy, my ill, my dying, and my miracle patients showed me what it looked like to be all of those things. Being a good studium, I took notes, I studied, and I learned from you. Then, when it was my turn and a life-defining moment punched me, I was prepared; I punched back with the ammunition of honesty, strength, and patience I had saved up over the years. I, the docere, became pati, and I got the chance to be just like you.

Full Circle:
The Survivor Lap

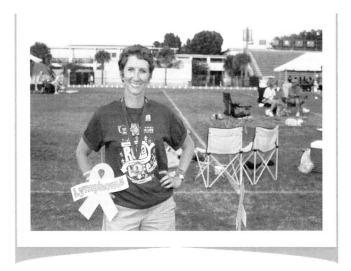

Photo by Shane Johnson

At the Brave's track for my first Relay for Life.

RX: Look for meaning. My guess is, you won't
have to look far. Life is providential that way.

The day after I found the mass on my chest x-ray, I took care of a patient I had originally met at a Bed, Bath, and Beyond store where she worked. In her workplace, she was friendly and helpful, and she had gone out of her way to make my shopping experience a delightful one. Since both of us worked in customer service arenas, we connected on a heart level through understanding and appreciating what customer service excellence looked like and felt like. Anyway, the May I found the mass in my chest, she came into my clinic with allergy and sinus symptoms. I already knew in that moment I saw her that my life was changing forever…I had seen the elephant. I was quietly scared and saddened that I may never see this kindred spirit again. In reality the picture was bigger than this, bigger than her spirit alone. I was grieving my own temporarily bruised spirit and wondering if I would even live through this tumor in my chest to see or to care for any patient ever again.

Now, fast forward one year to the next May. I was done with my treatments and I could breathe again. My port was gone. I went shopping for a new shower curtain to match some new luxuriously soft, chocolate-brown and celadon-green towels for a guest bathroom in my house. While standing in line at Bed, Bath, and Beyond, a manager was called to the checkout to help another customer, and who should begin her familiar walk to the front of the store? An expert in customer service, my patient, and a kindred spirit! She recognized me immediately and called out, "Hey, I know you!"

This was followed by a polite, "You cut your hair!" She hugged me. Right then and there in front of linens, towels, and shower curtains, I was compelled to share a short version of my story. As I did, a scale fell from my eyes, and I was stripped down to the beginning of this circle. In the same breath, I was at the end of the roundness. I was cleansed. I was going to be okay. *I am okay*, I thought to myself. I have made it full circle to look into the eyes of this kindred spirit that I wasn't sure I was going to ever see again. In her stark humanness, I suddenly became acutely aware of the past 365 days in my life and the love surrounding me. Life and love had been in the circle all along.

Life seems to always come full circle. Inside of the big circle of life, we are privileged to have many smaller full circles, and sometimes spirals, that either provide closure or seem to go on around one more time: ends that chase the beginnings again.

Every way I turned, it seemed other things also came full circle in the year after the storm. For example, simply said, my port went in, then my port came out. I had cancer. I didn't have cancer. I was the doctor who became the patient and then the doctor again.

I was living out my story after cancer, and I again saw one of the patients who had taught me to be a good patient! It was Jason, the melanoma survivor, who had seen me for a cough and a sore throat at my clinic several years ago and taught me a lesson in patience! He came back to our outpatient medical center for another sore throat and walked out a blessed hero after

I thanked him profusely for his life lesson. Seeing him again healed me yet again in the way that only blessing another life seems to do.

In yet another circle story, at a concert the weekend before the big crack I heard Mandisa Hundley, ninth place finalist in season five of *American Idol,* sing "Voice of a Savior." I didn't hear her voice for one full year, and then I was in my car on my way to a Relay for Life benefit for cancer, and her voice crooned on the car radio, "We'd give anything to hear…the voice of a Savior!"

At the Relay, I then walked in circles. Every year, in every major city, in almost every state and in sixteen other countries around the world, the American Cancer Society sponsors an all night walking event called the Relay for Life. The Relay benefits cancer research, pays for mammograms, and raises cancer awareness. Walkers are part of designated teams, and because cancer doesn't sleep, neither do the walkers. My first Relay for Life landed serendipitously on the anniversary weekend of the discovery of my cancer. My head full of a year of "I can't believe this was real" memories, the sometimes inexplicable tenacity of life, and wonder of the future, I drove to Boone High School in Orlando, "Home of the Braves," (how remarkably fitting) to walk as many circles around the track I could.

When I arrived at the oval track and field, I was already full of emotion, and I was amazed at the number of brown and green camping tents, event and food booths, and the number of people in the community that came out to support the event. The smell of barbecue and popcorn wafted in the sticky evening air. A fellow survivor handed me a purple survivor event T-shirt, a pin, and a ribbon. As the evening began, each one of us in purple shirts took center stage for a moment, introduced ourselves over a loudspeaker, named our diagnosis, and said how long we had been cancer free. We were each given a medal to wear over our heart—my first medal: a badge of honor and courage, just like a real warrior!

In a sea of purple, we survivors lined up at the start line and held hands. *Pufffft!* The sound of the race gun fired off, and hand-in-hand with other cancer survivors, I put one foot in front of the other and walked the lap of my life, the Survivor Lap. The sun was shining on us, and all of our family, friends, and supporting community stood on the infield and cheered and clapped as we took bold steps forward around the track. I felt like a hero—like I was back from a war. I had battled, was torn open, and now I was back in neutral territory! I was so proud to walk that lap! Volunteers sang, "Happy Birthday to You" as we walked and even passed out birthday cake!

For the second lap, our families walked with us. Hand in hand, Shane and I walked together, and with everyone else, we let out a collective sigh of relief. I walked my third lap with an eighty-five-year-old ovarian cancer survivor. She was short and spritely and attributed her longevity to growing up on a farm, milking the cows by age five, walking a mile and a half to and from school each day, and to living off the land her family farmed. After walking several laps past the bleachers and the goalposts around each bend, I felt like I was floating.

I stopped walking at one point and decorated white paper bag luminaries in honor of some members of the chemo posse and in memory of the one we lost. When it turned dark at the Home of the Braves, the luminaries were lit, and we all walked several laps to commemorate their lives. The luminaries lined the entire inner track and most of the outer track as well. In the bleachers, luminaries were lit that spelled out the word *H-O-P-E*. It was a beautiful sight to behold, but in my new eyes, there were too many candles, too many lives affected by this disease. Thank God for hope, but what is the reason for so many candles? What are we missing? Where do we go from here? Will there be answers in my lifetime? When will we come full circle?

Recovery Plan

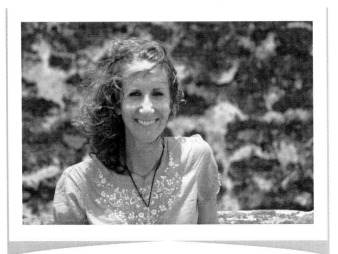

Photo by Shane Johnson

In San Juan, Puerto Rico two summers after treatment with a full head of new curly red hair.

RX: "Those who hope in the Lord will renew their strength. They will soar on wings like eagles; they will run and not grow weary, they will walk and not be faint" (Isaiah 40:31).

In an e-mail sent to the Army of Angels dated January 2 after I finished all of my treatments I wrote:

> Happy New Year! As many of you have gone through great trials this year as we have, we have certainly all come forth as gold. I, for one, am grateful for this year coming to an end, which marks the end of my seven-month battle against Hodgkin's lymphoma. I finished my last radiation dose on December 30th while I listened to "Superwoman" by Alicia Keys, "Celebration" by Kool and the Gang, and "Amazing Grace" by Ruben Studdard. As I lay on the hard radiation table as still as I could, the big, blue arm circling around me flashing its silver teeth, opening its jaws, humming and crackling away at me, I couldn't help but smile and think of the things that I have endured this past year.

I see now that cancer was not *in* the way, it was *the* way. As part of my recovery plan, I am coming to understand that as a survivor, I have some new obligations. Living through an interruption of my normal life not only has become an opportunity to live my life fuller, deeper, and through more focused eyes, but it also has become a responsibility for me to encourage (or to put courage into) others. In other words, cancer has become something I was given for the good of others. I realize now that my potential as a human is so much greater than just being a physician, a wife, a sister, a friend, and a daughter. I am an encourager, a prayer warrior, and someone who is not uncomfortable around the suffering of others.

During my illness, I became very aware that we are all suffering from something. They say that it takes a village to raise a child, yet I say that it also takes a village to raise up the wounded. I was blessed to be a part of the village on the receiving end, and I am honored to be a part of that village as a physician. I see my role in the village expanding, and I feel God moving my heart to give more from my heart, more from my past suffering. My pastor often says, "We lead through our strengths, but we connect through our weaknesses." Suffering can become one of our biggest weaknesses, or it can become one of our biggest strengths. We choose.

And when we see others suffering, we have yet another choice. How will we respond to them? Our suffering may appear individually vastly different on the outside yet is all the same at heart level. The heart is what connects us. Fighting through cancer or other illness, going through financial difficulty, losing a job, having a loved one die, or living in chronic pain are all days of suffering. Many wouldn't argue that. What they may argue about is whether there is an obligation that follows. As a human, I believe we do have an obligation of the heart to connect, to help ease the suffering of others, so we all may come forth as gold. In this simple act of comforting one another, we serve life.

I came forth as gold. I became fearless. I was inspired by Geneses 15:1, which says, "Do not be afraid…I am your shield, your very great reward." I have learned through my own suffering that being fearless doesn't merely mean the absence of fear. It means being afraid and going forward anyway. If you live fearlessly through faith, a punch of grace, a touch of humor, and perhaps an army of your own angels, I believe you will receive a hope and a promise of healing; and in doing so, you will transform your experience of suffering into a positive life discovery. You will be stronger, and ultimately, you will go on to recover in your own unique way.

A recovery plan is not written in a day; it is an ongoing process. For me, it meant walking around the block before I could run it. I had an opportunity to start over, to retrain. I had to learn on a conscious level what gave me energy and then I had to become intentional in how I used or conserved that energy. I learned what took my energy away and how to avoid those things or at least cut back on them. I learned to take a nap when I needed one instead of running "just one more errand!" I leaned on God more and leaned on myself less.

As I sit on my couch counting the years since I finished treatments, I still think about my cancer every day. I see my scars, and I am amazed at what my body went through in order to survive. I am thankful for the life force inside of me that built me into a survivor. When I reflect on my memories of that crazy, inexplicable year and the physical, emotional, and spiritual hurdles I jumped, all that I fought with and against, I am in awe. It is a lot. Although I sometimes feel that my healthy body betrayed me a few years ago, I have forgiven and I have overcome. I am filled with a spirit and a strength that was only on the surface before. I have deepened. The chemo may not be coursing through my veins any longer, but what it stands for—survival, healing power, instinct, lifeblood—is. I wear a new badge of honor and courage on my heart and in my soul. I am a survivor. I am fearless. I am healing.